About the author

Peggy Brusseau is an American who lives in London and teaches inter-disciplinary natural health education. She has written previous books about food and health, about the effect of movement on well-being, and regularly contributes articles to both popular health and professional healthcare journals.

A WI HELP YOURSELF GUIDE

Healthy Eating for Diabetics

Peggy Brusseau

CENTURY

LONDON · SYDNEY · AUCKLAND · JOHANNESBURG

First published in Great Britain in 1988 by
Century Hutchinson Ltd
Brookmount House, 62–65 Chandos Place,
Covent Garden, London WC2N 4NW

Century Hutchinson Australia (Pty) Ltd
89–91 Albion Street, Surry Hills,
New South Wales 2010, Australia

Century Hutchinson New Zealand Ltd
PO Box 40-086, 32–34 View Road, Glenfield,
Auckland 10, New Zealand

Century Hutchinson South Africa (Pty) Ltd
PO Box 337, Bergvlei 2012, South Africa

Set in 10pt Linotron Sabon
Printed and bound in Great Britain by
Mackays of Chatham Ltd, Chatham, Kent

British Library Cataloguing in Publication Data

Brusseau, Peggy
    Healthy eating for diabetics—(W.I.
    help yourself guide).
    1. Diabetics. Food – Recipes   2. Man.
    Diabetes
    I. Title   II. Series
    641.5'6314

ISBN 0-7126-2211-X

CONTENTS

Part One

Diabetes: What It Is and How It Happens

Living with Diabetes: Coping and Controlling

Part Two

Delicious Recipes for Diabetics

Part Three

Eating for a Good Life

What is the WI?

If you have enjoyed this book, the chances are that you would enjoy belonging to the largest women's organisation in the country – the Women's Institutes.

We are friendly, go-ahead, like-minded women, who derive enormous satisfaction from all the movement has to offer. This list is long – you can make new friends, have fun and companionship, visit new places, develop new skills, take part in community services, fight local campaigns, become a WI market producer, and play an active role in an organisation which has a national voice.

The WI is the only women's organisation in the country which owns an adult education establishment. At Denman College, you can take a course in anything from car maintenance to paper sculpture, from book-binding to yoga, or word processing to martial arts.

All you need to do to join is write to us here at the **National Federation of Women's Institutes, 39 Eccleston Street, London SW1W 9NT**, or telephone **01-730 7212**, and we will put you in touch with WIs in your immediate locality.

PART ONE

DIABETES: WHAT IT IS AND HOW IT HAPPENS

More than 30 million people around the world are known to suffer from diabetes. To give you some idea of that number, imagine that the total populations of London, Paris, Tokyo and New York are diabetic. And that is only the number of people who are *known* to suffer – perhaps as many people again are undiagnosed diabetics!

Anyone can suffer from diabetes, whether adult or child, but patterns are gradually emerging which indicate that this disorder is more common in those societies with Western diets and lifestyles. While this means that each one of us may be more likely than our Third World neighbours to develop diabetes, it may also mean that we can eventually minimize the number of people who develop diabetes by altering some aspects of our daily lives.

For those already living with diabetes, it is probable that greater diabetic control may be acquired in a similar way – by making a few simple changes in diet and lifestyle. But before we go into these changes, let's look at how this rather complex disorder affects nearly 2% of the Western population.

FROM DEFICIENCY TO DISORDER

There are several types of diabetes, but all derive from a deficiency of insulin or from an ineffective supply of insulin. Insulin is a hormone produced in the pancreas. Its job is to lower the level of glucose (sugar) in the blood. If, over a period of time, the quantity or quality of insulin production is impaired, then diabetes will almost certainly result.

Liver, Pancreas, Insulin and Glucose: How They Should Work
Diabetes manifests in the digestive process – in the way your food is metabolized. The whole point of digestion is to change food into its very basic parts so that your body tissues can derive nourishment from it. To begin this change, food undergoes a mechanical break down as in chewing, followed by a chemical break down – from the enzymes in your saliva, for instance.

This combination of mechanical and chemical action is continued throughout the digestive process. The mechanical actions are chewing, churning, squeezing and moving food through the digestive system. The chemical actions are performed by a variety of enzymes, each of which has a very specific effect upon your food. When talking of diabetes, look especially at the chemical action which occurs in the small intestine.

The contents of the stomach are passed by mechanical action into the small intestine, where digestion is continued. There, juices from the pancreas, the liver and the small intestine itself act on the partially digested food (chyme) to break it down further. The pancreas secretes enzymes which break down the fats and starches. The liver secretes bile which helps in the digestion of fats. And the small intestine secretes juices which further break down carbohydrates, fats and proteins.

As the food is digested its nutrients are absorbed, through the intestinal wall, into the blood stream and distributed throughout the body tissues. Fat and carbohydrate provide sources of energy, while protein builds and repairs protein tissues such as muscle. Any excess fat or protein which your body digests is stored in your body as fatty tissue. Any excess carbohydrate is also stored as fat or in your liver as glycogen – but only after it has first been converted to glucose.

It is necessary for you to have a certain amount of glucose in your blood at all times because glucose is your main source of energy. The correct level of glucose in your blood is maintained by the action of two hormones, insulin and glucagon, secreted by the pancreas. Insulin lowers the level of glucose (sugar) in the blood by helping the body tissues to either use it or store it, as glycogen, in the liver. Glucagon, the other hormone, raises the level of glucose when necessary by encouraging the liver to break down its stores of glycogen and release the resulting glucose into the blood. Together these two hormones maintain a minimum degree of fluctuation in blood sugar level . . . in a healthy person.

When Something Goes Wrong

Glucose is the final product in the digestion of carbohydrates and is the main source of energy to your body tissues. After a meal, it is natural to experience a rise in blood sugar level as your food is broken down into glucose. This is the time when insulin should begin its work of lowering the level of glucose in your blood by converting it to energy. However, some people do not produce enough insulin or else the insulin they produce does not function in the way it should. In these people, blood sugar rises to a very high level and eventually spills out into the urine signalling the onset of diabetes mellitus (the literal meaning of the word diabetes is 'sweet leakage').

With this shortage of insulin, glucose is not being converted to energy as it should be. And although the blood is full of glucose, none is reaching the body tissues. Recognizing a shortage of energy is one of the jobs of the liver and so it begins to convert its stores of glycogen into more glucose – thinking it will be converted to energy for the body tissues. However, the shortage of insulin prevents *this* glucose being converted to energy also. Instead the liver has added *more glucose* to an already overloaded bloodstream and so *more glucose* spills out into the urine!

At this point the body is still drastically short of energy and so it begins to break down its stores of fat and protein (muscle tissue) as the next step in supplying the body's needs. You can see the problem becoming more complex. As the body breaks down fat and protein, *more* glucose is produced and pushed into the bloodstream! If the supply of insulin is very low then, at this point, the diabetic is in real danger, because as the fats break down, substances called ketones appear in the blood and then in the urine. Ketones are the waste by-products of the breakdown of fats and in small amounts are not necessarily dangerous. However, in large amounts the ketones are acid and they can create a state of keto-acidosis: also called diabetic coma.

Many diabetics (non-insulin dependent) need not worry about the possibility of going into a diabetic coma because they produce just enough insulin to prevent the breakdown of body fats and proteins. However, those who are insulin dependent must avoid ketosis – the production of ketones in the blood and urine – by taking insulin well before this state is reached.

DIABETES MELLITUS: SYMPTOMS, CAUSES AND EFFECTS

The main symptoms of diabetes are excess urination and the presence of glucose in the urine. In fact, testing the urine for glucose is one way of knowing whether diabetes has developed. The level of glucose in the blood is the real issue, however, because the kidneys can deal with a certain amount of excess blood sugar and so prevent any glucose showing in the urine for a short period of time (1 – 2 hours). Once this 'renal threshold' has been surpassed, glucose appears in the urine, often well after a significant rise in blood sugar level has been experienced.

The frequency and volume of urine passed causes additional symptoms including feelings of thirst, hunger and weakness. In some people, itching of the genitals and a blurring of vision also accompany a high blood sugar level. In non-insulin dependent diabetes these symptoms need not appear all at once, nor all to a very noticeable degree. In insulin dependent diabetes, however, the symptoms may appear quite rapidly and distinctly. An additional symptom of sudden weight loss is usually experienced, due to the conversion of fat and protein tissues. Some unfortunate people experience a diabetic coma before their diabetes is diagnosed. Insulin is then necessary to save life.

Causes

The cause of diabetes is unknown. In some people an inherited trait increases their chances of developing the more severe, insulin dependent, type of diabetes. Stress in the form of acute trauma, infection or excessive drug usage may also initiate diabetic symptoms which may be temporary in adults, or more severe and perhaps permanent in children. A history of obesity, poor diet and lack of exercise may further provide the necessary conditions for diabetes to occur – especially in adults.

Maturity Onset Diabetes: Non–Insulin Dependent

'Overfed, overweight and underactive . . . ' That is a popular summary of many, but not all, adults who develop diabetes in their middle years. Maturity onset diabetics experience the basic symptoms of thirst, fatigue, hunger and frequent urination. However, their health may improve by losing weight, increasing their level of exercise and monitoring food intake to avoid foods high in calories, fats and sugar. In some people, diabetic symptoms may actually disappear following a strict regime of dietary control and exercise. Others must live the rest of their lives with the precautions, medications and attention to diet which have for so long been associated with the disorder. In maturity onset diabetes, the adult need not become insulin dependent.

Juvenile Onset Diabetes: Insulin Dependent

Although any age of person may develop diabetes, those who develop diabetes under the age of 40 years are most likely to suffer the more severe, insulin dependent, form. Children who develop diabetes are almost always insulin dependent.

The insulin dependent diabetic produces very little or no insulin and so relies on insulin injections. Without a supply of insulin he or she would not survive.

Onset of Diabetes in Pregnancy

The natural hormonal changes which a woman undergoes in pregnancy may cause her to experience changes in her ability to metabolize food. For some women (approximately 1 – 3%) pregnancy impairs their ability to tolerate glucose and they may, especially in their third trimester, display some of the signs of diabetes. This type of diabetes is often called 'gestational diabetes' and it commonly disappears shortly after the delivery of the child.

Many factors determine the severity of gestational diabetes including family history, the weight of any previous children, the woman's own weight and, predictably, the diet of the woman. All pregnant women benefit from a high fibre, low fat diet – but those whose diabetes is gestational may benefit even more in that they reduce the likelihood of having to take insulin during this time.

Effects

In long term diabetics, whether insulin or non-insulin dependent, health may gradually deteriorate in other ways. For instance, kidney problems, heart and circulatory disorders and liver dysfunction may manifest in later years. This is because when a deficiency of insulin occurs, other body functions are placed under stress. The body tissues may be deprived of nourishment due to the blood sugar spilling out into the urine rather than being absorbed into the body. For long term diabetics, a diet and lifestyle aimed at prevention and minimization of these errors is recommended.

LIVING WITH DIABETES: COPING AND CONTROLLING

Diabetes is controlled with a combination of drugs, diet and changes in lifestyle such as exercise and attitude.

DRUGS

Insulin dependent diabetics must take insulin in order to survive, but they must also attend to their diet and level of exercise to ensure that their insulin injections remain effective.

Non-insulin dependent diabetics may be able to control their diabetes through diet alone, but many take drugs as well. The most commonly used drug is a Sulphonylurea tablet which stimulates the pancreas to produce more insulin. A less often used drug is the Biguanide (Metformin) tablet which decreases the body's tendency to form glucose from muscle and fatty tissue, rather than from carbohydrates as it should. Some non-insulin dependent diabetics take both of these drugs.

EXERCISE & WEIGHT CONTROL

If you are diabetic and overweight, reducing your weight will enable you to control your diabetes more effectively: by keeping your blood sugar low if you are not insulin dependent, by enabling you to use smaller doses of insulin if you are insulin dependent. A carefully planned diet – low in fat, sugar and protein, but high in vitamins, minerals, fibre and complex carbohydrates – will help you begin to lose weight.

Once you have 'got to grips' with your dietary changes and needs, you can begin an exercise programme, or continue your favourite sport. Exercise helps you lose weight and improves your overall health and metabolism so that insulin acts more efficiently.

Controlling your body weight and maintaining good fitness are important aspects of diabetic control. They reduce the stress and work your body has to deal with. They also help you to 'cope' with the changes in lifestyle which your diabetes may require. You will feel better about yourself and you'll look and feel more attractive.

ATTITUDE & LIFESTYLE CHANGES

Accepting that you have diabetes is the first and most important change that must occur when you are first diagnosed as diabetic. This may be easier said than done but, if you can accept it, you may find it easier to enjoy your life and 'get on with it' in the way that you used to. Unfortunately, some people do not fully accept the change in their health and many of them, as a result, ignore their body's special needs. This may mean that they put themselves and those near to them through the unnecessary stress and upset of mood swings, hypoglycemia, or even diabetic coma.

Think again of those 30 million people who are known to have diabetes. Most of them live a full and happy life, many are famous, many more are very successful in their home and career. A few have proved that diabetes need not prevent one from climbing mountains, entering a triathlon or becoming the local squash champion. These people have 'conquered' their diabetes through their attitude to life. They have looked beyond the inconveniences of their disorder and have grasped opportunities to live their life to the full.

Diabetes does require practical changes, too. Apart from the use of insulin or tablets, a diabetic needs to establish a good diet and very regular eating patterns to prevent great fluctuations in blood sugar levels. For most diabetics, that means always having a high carbohydrate snack on hand and anticipating changes in blood sugar before they occur. Ideally, diabetics should wear or carry a card identifying their specific needs so that, in the event of their having a hypoglycemic attack, they may be treated by those near them.

DIET: WHAT YOU NEED & WHAT YOU SHOULD AVOID

Part of the treatment of diabetes, which is common to all forms, is a recommended change in dietary habits. The specific recommendations made by doctors and dieticians have changed drastically over the years. Earlier recommendations for a high protein, high fat, low carbohydrate diabetic diet, have been replaced by advice to eat a high complex carbohydrate (high fibre), low fat diet. This diet is proving much more healthy than its predecessor.

A high fibre (complex carbohydrate) diet reduces the after-meal surge in blood sugar level commonly experienced on a high fat, high sugar (simple carbohydrate) diet. This means that less insulin is needed, so doses may be reduced and problems with hypoglycemia are minimized.

A bonus side effect of this diet is that the disorders and diseases often associated with diabetics – such as obesity, hypertension, heart disease – are improved. In fact, the high fibre, low fat diet is one which is currently being recommended to the whole population – you probably know someone already who has improved his or her health by changing to more natural and 'whole' foods.

Now, further dietary changes are afoot, to do with fats and proteins and, more specifically, with animal fats and proteins. Long term studies of thousands of people are showing that animal products may not be doing us all that much good. In fact, for some people they might be downright deadly. Further studies must be completed to confirm scientifically without doubt that a diet free from animal products is healthier than a meat-based diet: that it would eliminate or greatly minimize one or more of our society's major diseases.

But why wait? Millions of people all over the world already live long, robust and healthy lives without eating animal fats and proteins. These people also have a substantially lower risk of developing diabetes ... coincidence? The answer may have to wait for another two or three decades (the time it takes to complete an epidemiological study of the necessary proportions). You, however, can adopt a diet low in or free of animal products now.

A diet low in animal products is safe, healthy, beneficial, fulfils all your nutritional requirements and may reduce the complications so often associated with diabetes. It is also so delicious you'll have no trouble avoiding the foods that can create problems for diabetics. And if you are concerned about the long-term health of your children, this diet may help to reduce greatly their risk of ever developing diabetes in the first place.

This book is based on high fibre, low fat diet recommendations and also avoids flesh foods. Although some recipes include dairy products, these comprise less than 25% of the recipes listed. Of these, all but two can be altered to avoid the use of dairy products (see Dairy Products, page 22).

A CONFERENCE OF NUTRIENTS

Selecting foods to match your special dietary needs is really an opportunity for you to learn more about the basics of nutrition. It is a fascinating subject and one that will easily become a part of your everyday life. Here is some introductory information. Further reading suggestions are listed at the end of the book.

Protein: Protein is made from amino acids. It enables the formation of all the body's tissues and has an essential role in the development of blood, hormones, antibodies and enzymes. As an adult, protein only needs to make up between 25% and 30% of your total calorie intake. That is probably a lot less than you are taking at the moment.

Protein is present in every living thing and it is very easy to obtain enough to maintain good health. Some excellent sources of protein are whole grains, beans (especially soybeans and soybean products), and seeds. Eaten in combination with fruits and vegetables, these foods provide a 'complete protein' meal —one that includes all the essential amino acids.

Fat: It is always wise to limit your intake of fats and this is especially so in diabetes when too much fat in your diet may contribute to heart and artery disease. High fat foods can also make you feel 'full' and so limit your consumption of more nourishing foods. Far better to rely on the 'hidden' fats in natural, whole foods, and to enjoy the occasions when you do use oils – as in salad dressings or vegetable sautés. Try to use oils high in linoleic acid, such as sunflower, soybean, corn or safflower.

Carbohydrate: Carbohydrates are either simple or complex. Simple carbohydrates are found in such foods as sugar, honey and some fruits. These carbohydrates provide instant energy because they are very quick and easy to digest.

Complex carbohydrates, or starches, are found in vegetables, fruits, grains, seeds and nuts. The conversion of complex carbohydrates into glucose occurs gradually, even slowly, and prevents the 'slump' so often felt when a quick burst of energy runs out. Instead, a steady supply of glucose is released into the bloodstream. Whole grains, fruits and vegetables are the best sources of carbohydrate for anyone, but are particularly important for the diabetic. Carbohydrates also contain cellulose, or fibre, which is indigestible but beneficial to health.

Fibre: This is the part of foods which the body cannot digest. It is important to digestion because it helps the intestine to function correctly. A high fibre diet slows down the digestive process. More nutrients are therefore taken from the food and the breakdown of food into glucose is more gradual, thus avoiding such great surges in blood sugar levels. Fibre also absorbs water which keeps the food moist and eases its passage through the bowel. Low fibre diets are associated with cancers of the bowel, colon and rectum, heart disease, obesity and varicose veins. A diet high in complex carbohydrates is naturally high in fibre.

Vitamins: Vitamins are organic substances found in all living things. They are necessary for growth and maintenance of health throughout one's life. Vitamins do not supply energy, they contain no calories, but they are essential for the proper functioning of all the body's systems. Most vitamins are available only through the diet.

There are two basic forms of vitamin: water-soluble and fat-soluble.

Water-soluble: These vitamins are easily lost in cooking, cutting, ageing and washing of the particular food. They are not stored in the body and so they must be taken daily if the recommended requirements are to be met. Any excess supplied to the body is excreted.

B-COMPLEX: This is a group of vitamins (B1, B2, B3, B6, B12, Folic Acid, Biotin, PABA, etc.) necessary for the healthy functioning of all your body's systems. Your metabolism of food relies heavily on these vitamins and a shortage will leave you feeling – and looking – dull, dry and nervous.

You can greatly increase your intake of the B group by adding whole grains, dark green leafy vegetables, seaweed, miso or yeast products to your diet. For instance, use kelp or kombu in soups and stews, miso as a spread on toast, bran or oats in your breakfast cereal and brewer's yeast in your salad dressings.

VITAMIN C: This vitamin is present in most fresh fruits and vegetables – especially citrus fruit, green peppers, broccoli and tomatoes. It helps in the absorption of all the vitamins and minerals in your diet and is essential in the maintenance of protein tissues. Vitamin C also strengthens the blood vessels, helps in all healing processes and may help to prevent infection and allergy.

Fat-soluble: These vitamins are lost in heat, light, air and cooking. They are stored in the fatty tissues of your body and so excess doses may cause toxic reactions.

VITAMIN A: Available in spinach, broccoli, carrots, and other dark orange or dark green vegetables, this vitamin is used in the growth and repair of skin and mucous membrane. It is necessary to the digestion of proteins and helps develop good teeth, bones and blood.

VITAMIN D: This vitamin is crucial in the absorption of calcium and the formation of bone tissue. It also helps to maintain blood clotting and healthy heart function. Vitamin D is one of the few vitamins which does not necessarily come from the diet – it may be formed from the effects of sunlight on the skin.

VITAMIN E: Present in nuts, olive oil, wheat germ and soya beans, this vitamin is an antioxidant and so helps to prevent the breakdown of substances in the body. It improves healing, blood flow, fertility, and the body's ability to withstand pollutants.

VITAMIN F: This vitamin consists of unsaturated fatty acids and it must be found in the diet because the body cannot manufacture the essential unsaturated fatty acids. The best sources of these fatty acids are the vegetable and seed oils, such as soybean and safflower. These are useful additions to the diet – as substitutes for saturated fat products. Vitamin F assists in the transport and effectiveness of the other fat-soluble vitamins. It is essential to the health of skin, arteries, thyroid and adrenal glands, mucous membranes and nerves.

Minerals: Minerals are needed to build and sustain the body. They are both organic and inorganic substances which must be taken in the diet. Every tissue in the body contains minerals and every bodily process and action requires minerals to be present in adequate supply. Minerals act together with other minerals and with vitamins. Mineral deficiencies not corrected by dietary changes are soon followed by illness.

CALCIUM: Calcium is most effective when taken with adequate amounts of vitamins A, C and D, and with Iron, Phosphorus and Magnesium. The healthy development of bones and teeth, as well as muscle and nerve tissues, depends on calcium intake. It is present in green leafy vegetables, molasses and milk products.

IODINE: An iodine deficiency can result in thyroid problems –which means disturbances in hormone production, metabolism, growth, speech and mental acuity. A deficiency is very easy to avoid if mushrooms or seaweeds (i.e. kelp and kombu) are included in your diet.

IRON: Get your supply of iron from dried fruits, dark green leafy vegetables and by cooking in an iron pot! Iron combines with protein in the body and, when further combined with copper, creates haemoglobin. Haemoglobin is the red colouring of your blood and is the transport system for oxygen to all your body tissues. Iron helps many of the vitamins and minerals do their work and builds your resistance to infection and disease.

MAGNESIUM: It is difficult to find a plant food that does not supply magnesium, but whole grains, seaweeds, nuts, dark green leafy vegetables and molasses are particularly good sources. This mineral helps convert glucose to energy and also helps in the breakdown of carbohydrate and protein. Magnesium must be present in order for the other vitamins and minerals to do their work.

PHOSPHORUS: This mineral is present in every cell in the body. It is an essential part of the metabolization of foods and it helps in the repair and maintenance of body tissues. Whole grains, beans and lentils, nuts and dairy products are rich in phosphorus.

ZINC: Yeast products, grains and seeds are tasty foods with useful quantities of zinc, though if you eat a variety of whole, unprocessed food, zinc will be present in greater amounts. Zinc is a component of insulin and plays an important role in digestion and the absorption of vitamins. Fertility, growth and healing are improved when sufficient zinc is taken in the diet.

HOW THEY WORK TOGETHER

Although certain foods are pointed out as excellent sources of one vitamin or mineral or another, a diet based on variety and in-season foods is a reliable way of ensuring that all the necessary nutrients are consumed. Some of the old standby meals are excellent examples of a fairly traditional response to this formula. Baked beans on toast and a cheese salad sandwich, for instance, both combine foods to obtain the maximum nutritional value from each of the meal's component parts.

Focus on the quality of the foods you purchase – freshness, naturalness, wholeness – and the methods you use to prepare them – raw, steamed, baked – to maximize the health giving characteristics of the food you select.

A DIABETIC'S CUPBOARD: FOODS TO INCLUDE

Fruits: Fresh fruits or fruit juices and unsweetened tinned and frozen fruits may be eaten by themselves or as part of a dessert, breakfast or beverage. Dried fruits, especially sun-dried, may be carried as a between-meals snack, used in sugarless cakes, in muesli or as a sweetener in savoury dishes.

Vegetables: Fresh, organic and in-season vegetables are the most nutritious and therefore most beneficial to health. They are a major component of salads, casseroles, soups and most savoury dishes. The preparation methods which help to retain the nutritional value of vegetables are those which use the vegetables raw, steamed, 'sautéd' in liquid, grilled and baked.

Grains, Legumes, Nuts & Seeds: These are the backbone of the meat-free diet in that they are available fresh all the year round and supply very basic nutritional needs in quantity. Foods from this group are best purchased whole and unprocessed. So, for instance, use brown rice instead of polished rice, raw nuts and seeds instead of roasted or salted, and all members of this food group organically grown if possible.

It is true that the foods in these first three groups are filling and bulky. After a few weeks, one becomes familiar with the quantities of food needed for a meal and about this time, too, one begins to notice changes in health and physical appearance. These first three food groups provide the high fibre, low fat features of your diet.

Dairy Products: If you use milk and eggs, it is worth purchasing low fat milk products and free range eggs. These are high protein foods, and often high in fat, so you do not need many of them.

However, if you do not generally use this group of foods, you may substitute non-dairy products for the milk and cheese included in a few of the recipes which follow. I recommend soya milk instead of cow's milk (soya milk is now available in most of the large supermarket chains). Instead of yoghurt, use soft tofu (soya milk cheese); instead of cottage cheese, use firm tofu. In recipes which include eggs, one tablespoon of tahini is often a good substitute when the egg is for binding purposes only.

A DIABETIC'S WASTE-BIN: FOODS TO AVOID

Fruits: Tinned, frozen or prepared fruits such as jams and fruit juices which have been sweetened should be avoided. Dried fruits which have been coated in sugar are not recommended, neither are candied fruits.

Vegetables: Those which have been over-cooked or stored too long are not going to be very nutritious and might as well be avoided for the fresh variety. Similarly, tinned, frozen or pickled vegetables that are dosed with sugar will rob you of nutrients and you would be better to avoid these products. Fortunately, recent consumer preferences have meant that most large supermarket chains have stopped buying these poor quality products.

Grains, Legumes, Nuts & Seeds: Highly refined products reduce the fibre content of your diet and should be avoided. Instead of white rice, eat brown; instead of white bread, eat whole wheat. Again, this is much easier of late, due to the supermarkets' compliance with consumer interests. Also, most towns have at least one shop that specializes in natural and/or whole foods if a product is not obvious in your local supermarket.

Dairy Products: Avoid high fat milk and cheese and minimize the number of eggs you consume. This becomes easier and more natural after a month or two of eating a high fibre diet.

Meat Products: Meat does not supply a broad range of nutrients, is generally high in fat and supplies no fibre whatsoever. Avoiding it creates more 'room' for the high fibre, low fat components of your diet *and* creates more opportunity for your health to improve.

Sugars & Fats: Both of these are essential parts of your diet and are present in much of the food you eat. But they are detrimental to health when they are eaten in quantity as highly refined extracts. Avoid refined sugars such as icing and caster sugar, use molasses, honey and fruit instead. Avoid saturated fats such as those contained in meat products, and using modest amounts of golden vegetable oils such as safflower, soya and corn. These contain vitamins which benefit your health.

CALCULATING THE COUNT

The recipes which follow are high fibre, low fat recipes. They are free of meat and minimize dairy products and refined foods. Each recipe has its carbohydrate and calorie count listed above its ingredients. These numbers have been *rounded up to the nearest 5*. To calculate the grams of carbohydrate or number of calories per serving, divide by the number of servings listed.

Most diabetics calculate their carbohydrate intake using the exchange system. This is the simple ratio of 10 grams of carbohydrate is equal to 1 exchange (10g CHO = 1 Exchange).

Many diabetics also watch their calorie intake, often dividing their total daily requirement between three meals and three snacks. The number of calories listed is a total for the dish and should be divided by the number of servings to arrive at calories per portion.

PART TWO

DELICIOUS RECIPES FOR DIABETICS

SOUPS

Red, White and Green Soup

SERVES 4
TOTAL CARBOHYDRATE: 50g
TOTAL CALORIES 525

115 g (4 oz) dried soy beans
2 medium sized onions
1 × 425 g (15 oz) tin of whole tomatoes
1.5 litres (2.5 – 3 pints) water
115 g (1/4 lb) chopped greens (spinach)
5 ml (1 tsp) freshly ground black pepper

Wash, soak, rinse and pressure cook the beans. Slice the onions and sauté in the tomato over a medium flame. Break the tomatoes as you stir the onions. Add the cooked beans to the tomato and onion sauté, then add the water. Stir often as you bring the mixture to a simmer. Wash and trim the greens. Drain the greens and add them to the bean mixture. Add the black pepper and simmer for a further 20 – 30 minutes. Serve hot or cold.

Hot Potato Soup

SERVES 4 – 6

TOTAL CARBOHYDRATE: 175 g

TOTAL CALORIES: 825

1 kilo (2 lb) potatoes
2 medium sized onions
15 ml (1 tbsp) yeast extract
5 – 10 ml (1 – 2 tsp) freshly ground black pepper
5 ml (1 tsp) caraway seed
1 – 2 litres (2 – 4 pints) of water
5 stalks of celery
3 bay leaves

Scrub and dice the potatoes then place them in a colander and rinse under cold water. Leave to drain. Peel and finely chop the onions. Sauté the onions in the yeast extract. Use a large, deep saucepan and stir constantly over a medium flame. When the onions are soft, add the potatoes, pepper and caraway seed. Stir well then add the water and keep stirring for 1 – 2 minutes. Bring the soup to a boil and simmer, covered, for 20 minutes. Wash and slice the celery and add to the soup. Add the bay leaves. Simmer for a further 10 – 15 minutes and serve.

Carrot & Chickpea Stew

SERVES 4 – 6
TOTAL CARBOHYDRATE: 130 g
TOTAL CALORIES: 730

170 g (6 oz) dried chickpeas
450 g (1 lb) carrots
3 cloves garlic (optional)
2 large onions
1 × 425 g (15 oz) tin of whole tomatoes
5 ml (1 tsp) freshly ground black pepper
1 – 1.5 litres (2 – 3 pints) water
1 strip of kombu (optional)
15 ml (1 tbsp) cider vinegar

Soak, rinse and pressure cook the chickpeas. Scrub the carrots
and slice in thin rounds. Peel and chop the garlic and onions.
Using a deep saucepan, sauté them in a little juice from the tin
of tomatoes. Add the ground pepper and carrots to the sauté
and stir well. Gradually add the tomatoes and water and bring
the mixture to a simmer. Add the kombu and the chickpeas
and stir. Simmer for 30 minutes. Just before serving, stir in the
vinegar.

Pea & Coriander Soup

SERVES 4
TOTAL CARBOHYDRATE: 120 g
TOTAL CALORIES: 650

225 g (8 oz) dried split green peas
1 litre (2 pints) water
1 strip of kombu (optional)
1 bunch fresh coriander
freshly ground black pepper to taste

Wash and drain the peas and place them in a deep saucepan. Add the water, cover and bring to the boil. Add the kombu and simmer for 45 minutes, stirring occasionally. Wash and pick over the coriander and chop it finely. Add the coriander and the pepper to the soup. Stir well and simmer for a further 15 minutes. Serve very hot with fresh bread.

Tangy Red Lentil Soup

SERVES 4 – 6
TOTAL CARBOHYDRATE: 105g
TOTAL CALORIES: 620

225 g (8oz) dried red lentils
1 litre (2 pints) water
25 g (1 oz) fresh coriander
1 medium sized fresh chilli
juice of 1 lemon

Wash the lentils very well, drain them and add the fresh water. Bring to the boil, then cover and simmer in a large saucepan. Wash and chop the coriander and the chilli. When the lentils have cooked for 10 minutes, add the chilli. Add the coriander 10 minutes later. Stir well and cook for a further 10 minutes (30 minutes in total) or until the lentils have completely lost their shape and are quite mushy. Stir in the lemon juice just before serving.

Rich Spinach & Onion Soup

SERVES 4 – 6
TOTAL CARBOHYDRATE: 90 g
TOTAL CALORIES: 645

450 g (1 lb) fresh spinach
450 g (1 lb) onions
3 cloves of garlic
10 ml (2 tsp) soya oil
2.5 ml (1/2 tsp) ground black pepper
570 ml (1 pint) water
15 ml (1 tbsp) margarine
5 ml (1 tsp) caraway seed
30 ml (2 tbsp) whole wheat flour
570 ml (1 pint) milk
2.5 ml (1/2 tsp) ground coriander

Wash, drain and slice the spinach into coarse strips. Thinly slice the onions and garlic. Heat the oil in a deep saucepan over a medium heat. Add the garlic and sauté until light brown, then add the onions. Stir well. Add the black pepper, spinach and water, reduce the heat and stir often.

In a small saucepan, melt the margarine and lightly sauté the caraway seeds. Sprinkle the flour over the margarine and stir constantly to make a roux. Keep stirring as you add the milk – a little at a time. Add the coriander to the sauce and stir until a smooth consistency is reached. Add the white sauce to the soup and stir very well.

Cook the soup for another 10 – 15 minutes, stirring often. Serve.

Sweet Corn Chowder

SERVES 4 – 6

TOTAL CARBOHYDRATE: 105 g

TOTAL CALORIES: 615

15 ml (1 tbsp) margarine
2.5 ml (1/2 tsp) paprika
15 ml (1 tbsp) whole wheat flour
570 ml (1 pint) milk
850 ml (1.5 pints) water
1 × 340 g (12 oz) tin of sweet corn
1 medium red pepper
1 medium green pepper

Melt the margarine in a large saucepan over a low heat. Stir
the paprika into the flour and sprinkle over the margarine. Blend
well into a thick paste, or roux. Mix the milk and water together
in a jug and gradually add to the roux, stirring all the time.
Add the sweet corn to the soup and simmer for 5 minutes,
stirring often. Wash and chop the peppers and add to the soup.
Stir well and simmer for a further 5 minutes. Serve immediately.

Swede & Carrot Soup

SERVES 4 – 6
TOTAL CARBOHYDRATE: 35 g
TOTAL CALORIES: 200

1 large swede
450 g (1 lb) carrots
1 litre (2 pints) water
5 ml (1 tsp) freshly ground black pepper
1 bunch of watercress

Peel and dice the swede. Scrub and chop the carrots. Add them
to the water in a deep saucepan and cook at a simmer for 20
minutes, or until they are tender.

Remove the pan from the heat and run the soup through a
hand mouli into another saucepan. Return the puréed soup
to the cooker, adding more water if necessary to give a
consistency you will enjoy. Stir well. Add the pepper and the
washed and chopped watercress. Stir well and bring the soup
to a simmer again. Serve immediately.

Cold Orange & Chestnut Soup

SERVES 4

TOTAL CARBOHYDRATE: 85 g

TOTAL CALORIES: 440

115 g (4 oz) *chestnut purée*
570 ml (1 pint) *water*
15 ml (1 tbsp) *soy sauce*
juice of 2 oranges
a pinch of cinnamon
225 g (8 oz) *plain yoghurt*

Measure the chestnut purée into a saucepan and gradually add the water, stirring constantly to avoid lumps. Place the mixture over a low flame and simmer gently for 10 minutes. Add the soy sauce to the soup and stir well. Squeeze the oranges and add the juice to the soup. Add the cinnamon and stir well. The soup should cook for a total of 20 minutes at a gentle simmer. Remove from the heat and allow to cool to tepid. Add the yoghurt and stir well. Pour into four soup bowls and chill before serving. If desired, a sprig of mint may be used as a garnish.

Watercress & Celery Soup

SERVES 4
TOTAL CARBOHYDRATE: 15 g
TOTAL CALORIES: 160

30 ml (2 tbsp) yeast extract
1.5 litres (3 pints) water
2 medium onions
5 ml (1 tsp) caraway seed
1 head of celery
1 bunch of watercress

Dissolve the yeast extract in the water. Pour 45 ml (3 tbsp) of this mixture into a deep saucepan. Place over a medium flame. Peel and thinly slice the onions then sauté them in the liquid. When the onions begin to soften, sprinkle the caraway seed over them and continue to sauté, stirring constantly. Add the rest of the water, stir very well and increase the flame to bring the broth to a gentle boil.

Meanwhile, scrub, trim and chop the celery. Wash, trim and chop the watercress. When the broth has boiled, add the celery and watercress. Stir very well, cover the pan and remove from the heat. Leave covered for at least 10 minutes before serving.

Broccoli, Barley & Banana Soup

SERVES 4
TOTAL CARBOHYDRATE: 105 g
TOTAL CALORIES: 490

115 g (4 oz) barley
1 litre (2 pints) water
2 ripe bananas
450 g (1 lb) broccoli
5 ml (1 tsp) freshly ground black pepper

Wash and drain the barley. Place in a deep enamel saucepan with the water. Stir well, cover the pan and bring the water to the boil. Reduce the heat and simmer the barley for 40 – 50 minutes or until quite tender. Peel then mash the bananas and add them to the cooked barley. Then put the soup through a hand mouli to break down the barley and give the soup an even consistency. Return the soup to the pan and place over a medium heat. If you wish for a more liquid soup, add a little more water at this stage.

Wash, trim and finely chop the broccoli and add to the soup. Stir in the broccoli and the black pepper, cover the pan and cook for 5 – 10 minutes longer. Serve immediately.

Cabbage & Carrot Soup

SERVES 4
TOTAL CARBOHYDRATE: 50 g
TOTAL CALORIES: 270

15 ml (1 tbsp) yeast extract
140 ml (5 fl.oz) water
2 medium onions
450 g (1 lb) carrots
450 g (1 lb) cabbage
1.5 litres (3 pints) water
2 bay leaves
freshly ground black pepper to taste
1 bunch of fresh parsley

Dissolve the yeast extract in the water then pour the mixture into a large, deep saucepan. Place the pan over a low flame. Peel and thinly slice the onions and sauté them in the yeast extract liquid. Stir often. When the onions are very soft, scrub, trim and shred the carrots and add them to the sauté. Stir often.

Wash and finely shred the cabbage and add to the onions and carrots. Stir very well and do not worry if the vegetables begin to stick to the pan. Add the rest of the water and turn up the flame. Stir the soup well, cover the pan and allow the soup to come to a low boil. Add the bay leaves and the black pepper, stir well and reduce the heat.

Let the soup simmer, covered, while you wash and chop the parsley. Stir the parsley well in, cover the pan and remove it from the heat. Allow it to sit for 5 minutes before serving.

SALADS

Potato Salad

SERVES 4
TOTAL CARBOHYDRATE: 90 g
TOTAL CALORIES: 395

500 g (1 lb) new potatoes
115 g (¹/4 lb) carrots
1 bunch of spring onions
2 – 4 sprigs of fresh parsley

Scrub and steam the potatoes until tender, then allow them to cool. Scrub and shred the carrots. Trim and thinly slice the onions. Wash and chop the parsley and mix all the ingredients together in a large salad bowl. Serve with a Yoghurt or Mustard Dressing (see Sauces and Dressings).

Pasta Salad

SERVES 4
TOTAL CARBOHYDRATE: 215 g
TOTAL CALORIES: 1085

225 g (8 oz) whole wheat pasta shells (gnocchi)
1 × 340 g (12 oz) tin of sweet corn
1 large green pepper
1 bunch of red radish
30 ml (2 tbsp) chopped chives or 2 spring onions

Cook the pasta, drain well and allow to cool. Empty the sweet corn into a large salad bowl. Wash and thinly slice the pepper, radishes and chives (or onions) and place them in the bowl along with the pasta and corn. Stir all together and serve with a Yoghurt or Mustard sauce.

Winter Roots Pickled Salad

SERVES 4
TOTAL CARBOHYDRATE: 50 g
TOTAL CALORIES: 230

2 large (approximately 450g/1 lb) raw beetroot
1 medium sized raw turnip
225 g (1/2 lb) carrots
1 medium onion
15 – 30 ml (1 – 2 tbsp) grated fresh ginger
285 ml (10 fl.oz) cider vinegar

Scrub and trim the beetroot, turnip and carrots and grate or shred them into a large salad bowl. Peel and thinly slice the onion and add to the salad. Grate the ginger and add to the salad. Stir the ingredients together and pour over the vinegar. Stir well and cover. Keep in a cool place for 1 – 4 hours. Stir again and serve with other salads or as a side dish to a hot meal.

Three Colour Salad

SERVES 4 – 6
TOTAL CARBOHYDRATE: 95 g
TOTAL CALORIES: 475

450 g (1 lb) 'beef' tomatoes
a little salt
1 × 340 g (12 oz) tin of sweet corn
1 small Cos lettuce
1 large red pepper
2 medium sized chicory

Wash the tomatoes and slice into wedges. Sprinkle a little salt over them, to remove any bitter flavour, and place to one side. Empty the sweet corn into a large salad bowl. Wash, drain and coarsely slice the lettuce, pepper and chicory and toss in with the corn. Drain the salt from the tomatoes and add them to the salad. Toss the salad gently and serve with your favourite dressing.

Radish & Butter Bean Salad

SERVES 2 – 4
TOTAL CARBOHYDRATE: 55 g
TOTAL CALORIES: 310

115 g (4 oz) dried butter beans
2 bunches of red radishes
1 bunch of spring onions
4 large sprigs of fresh parsley

Soak the beans overnight, rinse, drain and pressure cook for 20 minutes. Allow to cool. Wash the radishes, onions and parsley. Quarter the radishes, thinly slice the onions and chop the parsley. Stir together in a large bowl with the cooled beans. Add a dressing such as Mint Vinaigrette (page 88) and serve.

Black-Eyed Bean Salad

SERVES 4
TOTAL CARBOHYDRATE: 65 g
TOTAL CALORIES: 345

115 g (4 oz) dried black-eyed beans
1 bunch fresh coriander leaves
5 sticks of celery
50 g (2 oz) pimento
juice of 1 lemon

Soak the beans and the coriander separately in very cold water overnight. Rinse, drain and pressure cook the beans. Allow to cool. Wash the coriander and the celery and chop both quite finely. Add the pimento to the greens and stir together in a large bowl. Stir the cool beans into the mix then squeeze the lemon juice over all, stir again and serve.

Quick Autumn Salad

SERVES 4
TOTAL CARBOHYDRATE: 100 g
TOTAL CALORIES: 600

450 g (1 lb) of cooked kidney beans
225 g (¹/2 lb) carrots
¹/2 small head of white cabbage
2 medium sized oranges
25 g (1 oz) slivered almonds

Ensure the beans are fully cooked (if they are tinned, the label should say if cooking is necessary) and empty them into a large bowl. Scrub the carrots and shred them and the cabbage into the bowl. Peel the oranges well. Slice the oranges thinly then add the slices and any juice to the bowl. Stir the salad very well, sprinkle the almonds over the top and stir again gently. Serve with sauce or dressing if desired, although the orange juice may be sufficient for you.

Crunchy Salad

SERVES 4
TOTAL CARBOHYDRATE: 30 g
TOTAL CALORIES: 165

1/2 head of Cos lettuce
225 g (8 oz) sprouted mung beans
1 medium sized raw beetroot
3 small carrots
25 g (1 oz) fresh parsley

Wash and thinly slice the lettuce. Rinse the bean sprouts and allow them to drain. Scrub the beetroot and carrots and shred them. Wash, drain and chop the parsley. Toss all the ingredients together in a large salad bowl and serve with your favourite dressing i.e. Simple Lemon Dressing (page 89) or Simple Yoghurt Dip (page 89) are good with this salad.

Endive, Peppers & Onion Salad

SERVES 4
TOTAL CARBOHYDRATE: 10 g
TOTAL CALORIES: 105

2 sprigs of fresh mint
60 ml (2 fl. oz) cider vinegar
juice of 1 lemon
freshly ground black pepper to taste
225 g (8 oz) endive
1 medium green pepper
1 medium red pepper
1 bunch of spring onions

Wash the mint and chop very finely. Add it to the vinegar and lemon juice in a small jug. Stir together with the black pepper and put aside. Wash, trim and break the endive and place in a large salad bowl. Wash and chop the peppers – a fairly fine texture is nice in this salad. Trim the onions and slice them in thin rounds.

Mix all the ingredients together and pour the sauce over all. Stir gently and leave to sit for 10 – 15 minutes. Then toss it gently and serve.

Red Runner Salad

SERVES 4
TOTAL CARBOHYDRATE: 35 g
TOTAL CALORIES: 200

1 × 425 g (15 oz) tin of runner beans or freshly steamed runner beans
225 g (8 oz) sprouted mung beans
1 medium red pepper
115 g (¹/4 lb) button mushrooms
15 ml (1 tbsp) chopped fresh tarragon

Drain the runner beans and place in a large salad bowl. Rinse and drain the bean sprouts and add to the bowl. Wash the pepper and slice it into thin pieces and add to the salad. Clean the mushrooms and halve or quarter them. Add to the salad. Pick over the tarragon, chop finely and stir into the salad. Give the whole salad a hefty toss together and serve with lemon juice or the dressing of your choice.

Cucumber & Watercress Salad

SERVES 4
TOTAL CARBOHYDRATE: 20 g
TOTAL CALORIES: 240

3 cloves of garlic
2 spring onions
285 g (10 oz) plain yoghurt
1 large cucumber
freshly ground black pepper to taste
1 bunch of watercress

Peel the garlic and crush into a small bowl. Trim the onions and slice into thin rounds, including the green part, and add to the garlic in the bowl. Stir the yoghurt into the garlic and onion and allow to sit.

Wash the cucumber and chop it first into 2.5 cm (1 inch) rounds. Then slice each round into four or five strips. Use the whole cucumber and place the strips in a large salad bowl. Sprinkle the pepper over them and stir well. Wash the watercress and then chop coarsely. Add to the cucumber. Now add the yoghurt mixture to the large bowl and stir gently together. Serve immediately or chill for one hour before serving.

Mushroom, Ginger & Chicory Salad

SERVES 4
TOTAL CARBOHYDRATE: 25 g
TOTAL CALORIES: 160

25 g (1 oz) fresh grated ginger
juice of 1 lemon
450 g (1 lb) chicory
225 g (1/2 lb) mushrooms
1 eating apple

Grate the ginger into the lemon juice and stir them together. Wash and slice the chicory and place in a salad bowl. Clean and thinly slice the mushrooms and add to the chicory. Wash, quarter and core the apple and chop into fine pieces. Add to the chicory and mushrooms. Stir the ginger and lemon in with the salad and serve immediately.

Cucumber, Mint & Tomato Salad

SERVES 4

TOTAL CARBOHYDRATE: 40 g

TOTAL CALORIES: 235

900 g (2 lb) 'beef' tomatoes
a little salt
1 large cucumber
2.5 ml (1/2 tsp) freshly ground black pepper
10 ml (2 tsp) honey
140 ml (5 fl.oz) cider vinegar
4 small sprigs of fresh mint

Wash and slice the tomatoes and arrange on a plate. Sprinkle a little salt over them to remove any bitter flavour and place to one side. Wash and thinly slice the cucumber and arrange in layers in a broad, shallow bowl. Sprinkle a little pepper in between each layer. Mix the honey and vinegar together in a jug and pour over the sliced cucumber. Place to one side. Wash and finely chop the mint and place in a large salad bowl. After soaking for at least 10 minutes, add the cucumber and vinegar sauce to the mint and stir well.

Drain the tomatoes and serve two or three slices on a small plate, then top with the mint and cucumber salad. Make sure that each serving has a little extra vinegar sauce.

Very Green Salad

SERVES 4 – 6
TOTAL CARBOHYDRATE: 20 g
TOTAL CALORIES: 160

450 g (1 lb) fresh broccoli
1 bunch of watercress
1 small Cos lettuce
225 g (¹/2 lb) cabbage
2 large spring onions

Wash, trim and steam cook the broccoli. Allow to cool. Wash and finely chop the watercress and place in a large bowl. Wash and slice the lettuce and cabbage and add to the watercress. Wash, trim and thinly slice the onions and add to the salad. Add the cooled broccoli and stir together.

Serve with other salads or as a starter to a hot dish. Use the dressing of your choice, i.e. Mustard Sauce 2 (page 87), Mint Vinaigrette (page 88).

Gourmet Orange & Asparagus Salad

SERVES 4

TOTAL CARBOHYDRATE: 45 g

TOTAL CALORIES: 190

450 g (1 lb) asparagus
225 g (¹/₂ lb) runner beans
2 large carrots
1 bunch of radishes
1 large orange

Wash, trim and steam the asparagus and the runner beans (15 – 20 minutes). Allow to cool. Scrub, trim and shred the carrots and place in a large salad bowl. Wash, trim and slice or quarter the radishes and add to the carrots. Peel the orange and divide it into segments, then slice each segment in half and add to the bowl.

Stir the cooled asparagus and runner beans into the salad and serve with the dressing of your choice, i.e. Yoghurt Sauce 1, (page 87), Simple Lemon Dressing (page 89). This is an excellent light lunch.

All-Colours Spring Salad

SERVES 4
TOTAL CARBOHYDRATE: 85 g
TOTAL CALORIES: 880

450 g (1 lb) mangetout
225 g (¹/₂ lb) button mushrooms
1 medium red pepper
1 × 340 g (12 oz) tin of sweet corn
1 medium avocado
30 ml (2 tbsp) chopped, fresh parsley

Wash and trim the mangetout and steam them for approximately 4 minutes. Allow to cool. Clean and slice the mushrooms and red pepper and place in a large salad bowl. Add the sweet corn and the cooled peas. Peel and coarsely chop the avocado and add to the salad. Wash and finely chop the parsley and add to the salad. Stir the whole together very well and serve with the dressing of your choice, i.e. Mustard Sauce 2, (page 87), Yoghurt Sauce 1 (page 87), Fennel Sauce (page 91).

MAIN DISHES

Brassica Bake

SERVES 4
TOTAL CARBOHYDRATE: 50 g
TOTAL CALORIES: 430

1 large cauliflower
450 g (1 lb) broccoli
Sauce:
1 small onion
3 cloves of garlic (optional)
15 ml (1 tbsp) oil
15 ml (1 tbsp) whole wheat flour
285 ml (10 fl.oz) low fat milk
140 ml (5 fl.oz) water
1 small red pepper

Wash, trim and cut the cauliflower and broccoli into florets. Place them together in a deep casserole. Peel the onion and garlic and chop quite finely. Heat the oil in a saucepan and sauté the garlic first, then the onion. Add the flour to the sauté and stir into a thick paste. Gradually add the milk and water, stirring all the while to a smooth sauce. Wash and chop the pepper and add to the sauce. Stir well and pour over the brassica.

Cover the casserole and bake at 170°C/325°F/Gas Mark 3 for 30 minutes. Uncover and cook for a further 5 minutes. Serve immediately.

Spinach Sauce Over Rice

SERVES 4
TOTAL CARBOHYDRATE: 215 g
TOTAL CALORIES: 1045

225 g (8 oz) brown rice
570 ml (1 pint) water
Sauce:
1 large onion
270 ml (10 fl.oz) water
140 ml (5 fl.oz) tomato purée
10 ml (2 tsp) dried parsley
5 ml (1 tsp) dried basil
freshly ground black pepper to taste
450 g (1 lb) fresh spinach

Wash the rice three times, drain and cook in the water until
the water is completely absorbed. Peel and chop the onion and
sauté in a little of the water in a deep frying pan. Add the
tomato purée, the rest of the water, and the parsley, basil and
pepper to the onions. Stir well as you bring the mixture to a
simmer over a medium heat. Cover the pan and reduce the heat.

Wash and drain the spinach, trim and chop it coarsely. Pack
the spinach into the pan with the tomato sauce, cover once
again and leave untouched for 15 minutes over the low heat.
At the end of this time, stir the spinach into the tomato sauce
and leave over the low heat until the rice is cooked. Serve the
sauce over the rice on heated plates.

Cauliflower in Mustard Sauce

SERVES 4
TOTAL CARBOHYDRATE: 55 g
TOTAL CALORIES: 590

1 *large cauliflower*
2 *small onions*
Mustard Sauce 1 *recipe (page 86) using twice the amount of liquid*
50 g (2 oz) breadcrumbs
3 *cloves of garlic*
10 ml (2 tsp) sesame seeds

Wash the cauliflower and cut into florets. Peel and chop the
onions then stir together with the cauliflower into a deep
casserole dish. Make the Mustard Sauce and pour over the
cauliflower and onion mixture, stir well. Mix the breadcrumbs,
chopped garlic and sesame seeds together in a bowl then sprinkle
the mixture over the cauliflower.

Cover the casserole and bake at 170°C/325°F/Gas Mark 3
for 30 minutes. Uncover and continue baking for a further 10
minutes. Serve immediately with a green vegetable or a salad.

Rustic Baked Beans

SERVES 4 – 6
TOTAL CARBOHYDRATE: 90 g
TOTAL CALORIES: 1000

225 g (8 oz) dried soya beans
Rich Tomato Sauce recipe (page 85)

Wash, soak, rinse and pressure cook the beans. Make up the sauce. You may wish to double the quantity, depending on the richness and thickness of sauce you prefer. Add the cooked beans to the sauce and simmer together for at least 30 minutes.

This recipe improves with time. Serve alone, with Nutless Loaf or with baked potatoes. Excellent cold too, for picnics and packed lunches.

Italian Rice

SERVES 4
TOTAL CARBOHYDRATE: 185 g
TOTAL CALORIES: 860

225 g (8 oz) dried brown rice
570 ml (1 pint) water
Sauce:
1 × 455 g (16 oz) tin of whole tomatoes
2.5 ml (1/2 tsp) freshly ground black pepper
3 cloves of garlic (optional)
5 ml (1 tsp) dried parsley or 2 sprigs chopped fresh parsley
2.5 ml (1/2 tsp) dried basil

Wash and drain the rice and cook in the water. Mix the remaining ingredients together in a saucepan and simmer gently until the rice is cooked. Serve the sauce over the rice - this is a simple, high fibre dish and very quick to make.

Winter Layers Casserole

SERVES 4 – 6

TOTAL CARBOHYDRATE: 145 g

TOTAL CALORIES: 655

450 g (1 lb) potatoes
450 g (1 lb) parsnips
450 g (1 lb) carrots
1 large onion
5 ml (1 tsp) freshly ground black pepper
30 ml (2 tbsp) yeast extract
450 ml (³/4 pint) water

Warm the oven to 180°C/350°F/Gas Mark 4. Scrub the vegetables and peel the onion. If possible, use a food processor to save time and slice the vegetables and onion, keeping them separate. Place the vegetables in rough layers in a deep casserole: parsnip, carrot, potato, parsnip, etc. until they are all used. Sprinkle the ground pepper over the top layer and spread the onion slices over this. Mix the water and yeast extract together and pour over all. Cover the casserole dish and bake for 55 minutes.

Easy Dhal

SERVES 2 – 4
TOTAL CARBOHYDRATE: 115 g
TOTAL CALORIES: 695

225 g (8 oz) red lentils
570 ml (1 pint) water
3 cloves of garlic (optional)
2 small onions
1.25 ml (1/4 tsp) or 2.5 ml (1/2 tsp) chilli powder
1/2 bunch of fresh coriander

Wash the lentils very well, until the water that drains from them is clear. Add the fresh water to them and bring to a boil. Then cover the pan and simmer. Chop the garlic and onion very finely and sauté in 30 ml (2 tbsp) of water. Add the onions, garlic and chilli powder to the lentils and stir well. The smaller measure of chilli will yield a mild dhal, the larger measure a warming dhal. Wash and chop the coriander.

When the lentils have simmered for 20 minutes, stir the chopped coriander into the dhal and leave to simmer another 5 – 10 minutes. Serve over rice as a main meal, or as a soup or side dish.

Economy Marinade

SERVES 6 – 8
TOTAL CARBOHYDRATE: 75 g
TOTAL CALORIES: 635

The Marinade:
270 ml (1/2 pint) cider vinegar
juice of 2 lemons
12 whole cloves
12 whole peppercorns
5 ml (1 tsp) caraway seed
140 ml (5 fl.oz) apple juice
3 bay leaves
2 small pieces of cinnamon
270 – 450 ml (1/2 – 3/4 pint) water
The Vegetables:
225 g (1/2 lb) carrots
340 g (12 oz) runner beans (tinned or frozen)
1 small red pepper
1 small green pepper
2 small onions
1 medium sized cauliflower
450 g (1 lb) broccoli

Gently heat all the Marinade ingredients together in a large enamel saucepan while you prepare the vegetables.

Wash the vegetables. Thinly slice the carrots, beans, peppers and onions. Cut the cauliflower and broccoli into florets.

Simmer all the vegetables in the marinade for 15 minutes. Keep the pan covered but stir often. Then remove the pan from the heat and allow the mixture to cool. Serve immediately or keep chilled in the fridge for 3 – 4 days.

Tempeh Marinade

SERVES 4
TOTAL CARBOHYDRATE: 50 g
TOTAL CALORIES: 430

225 g (8 oz) tempeh
150 ml (5 fl.oz) cider vinegar
75 ml (2.5 fl.oz) soy sauce
5 ml (1 tsp) mustard seed
12 whole cloves
12 whole peppercorns
3 – 6 cloves of garlic (optional)
225 g (¹/₂ lb) onions

Defrost the tempeh and cut into 1-inch cubes. Place the tempeh in a casserole dish. Mix the vinegar, soy sauce and spices together in a jug. Finely chop the garlic and onions and add to the marinade. Stir well and pour over the tempeh pieces. Cover the casserole and leave the tempeh to marinate for 4 – 8 hours.

Bake, covered, at 170°C/325°F/Gas Mark 3 for 30 minutes. Remove the cover and bake for a further 10 minutes. Serve with brown rice and steamed broccoli.

Baked Pasta Shells in Creamy Tomato Sauce

SERVES 4

TOTAL CARBOHYDRATE: 200 g

TOTAL CALORIES: 1100

225 g (8 oz) whole wheat pasta shells (gnocchi)
225 g (1/2 lb) onions
3 – 6 cloves of garlic (optional)
10 ml (2 tsp) soya oil
140 g (5 oz) tomato puŕee
2.5 ml (1/2 tsp) each of dried basil, parsley, oregano and ground black pepper
350 ml (12 fl. oz) low fat milk
350 ml (12 fl.oz) water

Weigh the pasta and empty into a deep casserole. Chop the onion and garlic and sauté in the hot oil. Remove from the heat and add the tomato purée, herbs and pepper. Stir well, gradually adding the milk and water.

Pour the sauce over the pasta shells and bake at 180°C/350°F/ Gas Mark 4 for 45 minutes. Serve immediately.

Sweet & Sour Mushrooms over Spaghetti

SERVES 2

TOTAL CARBOHYDRATE: 95 g

TOTAL CALORIES: 505

1 medium sized onion
3 cloves garlic
30 ml (2 tbsp) vinegar
225 g (1/2 lb) button mushrooms
2 large prunes
15 ml (1 tbsp) brewer's yeast
5 ml (1 tsp) freshly ground black pepper
115 g (4 oz) whole wheat spaghetti

Chop onion and garlic and sauté in the vinegar in a large frying pan. Clean and thickly slice the mushrooms and add to the sauté. Stir in the prunes, yeast and pepper, blend well and simmer very gently while you cook the spaghetti. Serve the sauce over the spaghetti.

Mexican Tostadas

SERVES 6
TOTAL CARBOHYDRATE: 255 g
TOTAL CALORIES: 1220

12 *corn-meal tostadas*
1 Red Bean Paste *recipe (page 95)*
115 g *(¹/4 lb) carrots*
1 *medium sized beetroot*
1 *medium sized onion*
¹/2 *head of lettuce*
1 *bunch of fresh parsley*

Warm the tostadas in a hot oven for 2 – 3 minutes on a baking tray. Make the Red Bean Paste. Wash and prepare the vegetables and arrange them in separate dishes: grate the carrots and beetroot, slice the onion and lettuce and chop the parsley.

Prepare a sauce of your choice (i.e. Simple Yoghurt Dip or Very Own Catsup) or just use a squeeze of lemon juice.

Spoon a little bean paste on to each tostada and spread to the edges. Then sprinkle a little of each of the salad ingredients over the bean paste and finally top with a sauce, if desired. Serve cold.

Red Bean Curry

SERVES 4
TOTAL CARBOHYDRATE: 125 g
TOTAL CALORIES: 695

225 g (8 oz) dried red beans (kidney or pinto)
10 ml (2 tsp) oil
3 cloves garlic
2 small onions
5 ml (1 tsp) cumin
10 ml (2 tsp) yeast extract
300 – 400 ml (1/2 – 3/4 pint) water
1 fresh chilli or 1 small green pepper
5 ml (1 tsp) garam masala

Wash, soak, rinse and pressure cook the beans. Heat the oil in a frying pan and chop the garlic and onion. Sauté the garlic until brown and then add the onion. Add the cumin and stir well. Add the yeast extract and stir continuously as you add the water. Add the beans and mash them slightly. Cover the pan and allow the mixture to simmer for 10 minutes.

Meanwhile chop the chilli (if you want a hot curry), or the pepper (if you prefer a mild curry). Add to the mixture and stir well. Simmer, covered, for a further 10 minutes then stir in the garam masala. Remove the curry from the heat but leave covered for a further five minutes before serving.

Ladies' Fingers Savoury

SERVES 4
TOTAL CARBOHYDRATE: 20 g
TOTAL CALORIES: 190

450 g (1 lb) fresh ladies' fingers (okra)
3 cloves of garlic
2 small onions
15 ml (1 tbsp) yeast extract
140 – 200 ml (4 – 7 fl.oz) water
225 g (1/2 lb) button mushrooms

Wash the ladies' fingers and cut off the hard top of each one. Chop the garlic and onion and sauté in the yeast extract stirred into a small amount of the water. Add the ladies' fingers to the sauté and stir frequently over a high flame. Clean the mushrooms and add them to the sauté. Stir well and cook for another 3 – 4 minutes over the high flame. Add the remaining water to get the amount of gravy you desire. Cover and cook for 5 minutes longer. Serve immediately with rice, pasta or steamed vegetables.

Leek & Brussels Sprout Stir-Fry

SERVES 4
TOTAL CARBOHYDRATE: 35 g
TOTAL CALORIES: 245

450 g (1 lb) Brussels sprouts
225 g (1/2 lb) leeks
15 ml (1 tbsp) yeast extract
285 ml (10 fl.oz) water
10 ml (2 tsp) caraway seed
freshly ground black pepper to taste

Wash and trim the sprouts and leeks. Cut the sprouts in half
and slice the leeks into thin rounds. In a broad saucepan, heat
the yeast extract mixed with a small amount of water. Sauté
the caraway seed and the sprouts, stirring often. The sprouts
will begin to brown on the cut edges. Add the sliced leeks and
the rest of the water and stir constantly for 5 minutes over a
medium flame. Add the black pepper, stir and cover for a further
5 minutes cooking over a low flame. Serve immediately with
rice, pasta, baked potato or toast.

Scented Rice

SERVES 4 – 6
TOTAL CARBOHYDRATE: 180g
TOTAL CALORIES: 840

225 g (8 oz) brown rice
710 ml (1¹/4 pints) water
2.5 ml (¹/2 tsp) turmeric
5 ml (1 tsp) mustard seed
juice of 1 lemon

Wash and drain the rice. Bring the water to a low boil and add the turmeric. Stir well, then add the rice. Bring to a boil then simmer, covered, until the water is absorbed.

Coarsely crush the mustard seed and stir into the rice along with the lemon juice. Serve hot or cold with salads or steamed vegetables or a savoury dish.

Special Scented Rice

SERVES 4 – 6
TOTAL CARBOHYDRATE: 100 g
TOTAL CALORIES: 895

225 g (8 oz) brown rice
850 ml (1¹/2 pints) water
5 ml (1 tsp) turmeric
1 bay leaf
1 × 5 cm (2 inch) piece of cinnamon
1 small onion
285 g (10 oz) fresh or frozen peas
1 small red pepper
1 small green pepper

Wash and drain the rice. Bring the water to a low boil and add the turmeric, bay leaf and cinnamon stick. Stir well, then add the rice and bring to the boil again. Cover and simmer for 10 minutes.

Peel and finely chop the onion. Stir the onion and peas into the cooking rice and cover the pan once more. Wash and chop the peppers. Add them to the rice when the water is nearly all absorbed. Cover the pan and cook another 5 minutes, or until the rice is ready. Stir well and serve hot or cold with salads, vegetables or other savoury dishes.

Millet & Vegetable Pot with Olives

SERVES 4 – 6
TOTAL CARBOHYDRATE: 170 g
TOTAL CALORIES: 1070

1 litre (2 pints) boiling water
225 g (8 oz) dry millet
115 g (4 oz) pitted green olives
1 bunch of spring onions
1 bunch of watercress
1 bunch of radish
pinch of paprika

Bring the water to a hard boil and add the millet. Simmer for 20 minutes, covered. Drain the olives and cut each one in half. Wash, trim and slice the spring onions. Wash and chop the watercress and the radishes. Drain the millet and place it in a steamer lined with cheesecloth. Steam for 20 minutes.

Stir the prepared vegetables into the steamed millet and serve immediately with a sauce of your choice, or with salt and pepper.

Bulghur & Coriander Half-Bake

SERVES 4

TOTAL CARBOHYDRATE: 180 g

TOTAL CALORIES: 860

710 ml (1¹/4 pints) water
15 ml (1 tbsp) yeast extract
1 small onion
225 g (8 oz) bulghur wheat
28 g (1 oz) chopped fresh coriander

Measure the water into a deep saucepan and bring to the boil. Stir in the yeast extract until it is dissolved. Peel and finely chop the onion and add to the water. Add the bulghur wheat to the water, stir well and cover the pan. Cook over a low heat for 2 minutes. Wash and chop the coriander then stir it into the bulghur wheat.

Transfer the bulghur wheat to a casserole dish, cover and bake at 170°C/325°F/Gas Mark 3 for 20 minutes. Serve immediately with a little soy sauce if desired.

Nutless Hot 'n Cold Loaf

SERVES 4 – 6
TOTAL CARBOHYDRATE: 165 g
TOTAL CALORIES: 855

55 g (2 oz) red lentils
2 packets of No-Salt VegeBurger dry mix
55 g (2 oz) rolled oats
2.5 ml (1/2 tsp) chilli powder
10 ml (2 tsp) dried parsley
400 ml (14 fl.oz) water
Sauce:
30 ml (2 tbsp) tomato purée
140 ml (5 fl.oz) water
5 ml (1 tsp) mixed sweet dry herbs

Wash and drain the lentils. Stir the dry ingredients together in a mixing bowl. Add the lentils and the water and stir very well. Leave to sit for 10 minutes.

Lightly oil a loaf tin and warm the oven to 170°C/325°F/Gas Mark 3. Make the sauce by mixing the tomato, water and herbs together. Stir the loaf mixture once again and press into the loaf tin. Bake for 10 minutes then remove from the oven and pour the sauce over the loaf. Cover the tin with foil and return to the oven. Bake for 40 minutes. Serve hot with vegetables, or cold sliced into sandwiches.

Aduki Bean & Bamboo Shoot Savoury

SERVES 4
TOTAL CARBOHYDRATE: 85 g
TOTAL CALORIES: 520

115 g (4 oz) dry aduki beans
570 ml (1 pint) water
1 × 285 g (10 oz) tin of bamboo shoots
1 bunch of spring onions
60 ml (2 fl.oz) water
freshly ground black pepper to taste.

Wash, pick over and drain the beans. Cover them in the water and bring to the boil. Cover the pan and simmer for 45 – 60 minutes, or until soft. Rinse the bamboo shoots under cold water and drain. Wash and trim the onions and slice along their length to include the green portion.

When the beans are nearly cooked, place the bamboo shoots, onions and the small measure of water in a frying pan over a medium flame. Stir continuously for about 5 minutes. Drain the beans and add them to the bamboo and onion mix. Add the pepper and stir the whole gently together. Serve over rice, pasta or with other vegetables.

Sweet Potato Bake

SERVES 4
TOTAL CARBOHYDRATE: 90 g
TOTAL CALORIES: 400

450 g (1 lb) sweet potatoes
1 large orange
2.5 ml (¹/₂ tsp) freshly ground black pepper

Scrub the sweet potatoes and quarter them, cutting only three quarters of the way through so that you are able to open them. Lay each potato on a piece of foil or arrange them together in a large baking tray. Peel the orange, divide it into segments and cut each segment in half. Place the orange pieces in the centre of each 'open' potato. Sprinkle a little black pepper over each potato.

Wrap or cover the potatoes and bake at 180°C/350°F/Gas Mark 4 for 45 minutes. Serve immediately with other vegetables and your favourite sauce.

Hot Arame & Broccoli Salad

SERVES 4

TOTAL CARBOHYDRATE: 35 g

TOTAL CALORIES: 120

50 g (2 oz) arame seaweed
water to cover
450 g (1 lb) broccoli
1 bunch of spring onions
60 ml (2 fl.oz) soy sauce

Rinse the arame then soak it in a bowl of cold water for 5 minutes. Move the arame around in the water to free any particles of sand, then lift out of the water and drain. Throw the water away.

Place the arame in a saucepan and cover with water. Cover the pan and bring the water to the boil. Reduce the heat and simmer for 20 minutes.

Wash and trim the broccoli then steam it for 10 – 15 minutes or until tender. Wash and trim the onions and slice into thin rounds.

When the arame has cooked, drain the water from it and add the broccoli and onions. Stir them together, then add the soy sauce. Place over a medium flame for 5 – 10 minutes, stirring occasionally. Serve immediately with a little black pepper. This is delicious with rice or other vegetables.

Carrot & Spring Onion Sauté

SERVES 4
TOTAL CARBOHYDRATE: 20 g
TOTAL CALORIES: 220

3 cloves of garlic
10 ml (2 tsp) oil
450 g (1 lb) carrots
1 bunch of spring onions

Peel and chop the garlic and sauté in the oil. Scrub and trim the carrots then slice them into thin rounds. Add them to the sauté and stir frequently. Wash and trim the onions and slice thinly along their length. Add them to the sauté, leaving them on top of the carrots.

Cover the pan and reduce the heat. Leave covered for 10 minutes then remove the cover, stir the sauté well and serve with rice, Nutless Hot 'N Cold Loaf, (page 69) or other vegetables.

Spinach & Chickpea Savoury

SERVES 4
TOTAL CARBOHYDRATE: 100 g
TOTAL CALORIES: 675

170 g (6 oz) dry chickpeas
450 g (1 lb) fresh spinach
15 ml (1 tbsp) yeast extract
100 ml (4 fl.oz) water
3 cloves garlic
2 medium onions
2.5 ml (1/2 tsp) freshly ground black pepper

Wash, soak and cook the chickpeas. Wash trim and drain the spinach. Mix the yeast extract in the water and pour a small amount in a deep frying pan or saucepan. Place over a medium flame.

Peel and chop the garlic and sauté in the yeast gravy. Add the onion and continue to sauté, stirring frequently. Add the cooked chickpeas and the black pepper to the sauté and stir well. Cover the sauté for about 5 minutes.

Roughly slice the spinach and place on top of the chickpeas. Cover the pan again and leave over a low flame for 10 – 15 minutes. Do not remove the cover. At the end of this time, stir the spinach into the chickpeas and serve immediately by itself, with rice or steamed vegetables.

Mexican Chilli

SERVES 4
TOTAL CARBOHYDRATE: 100 g
TOTAL CALORIES: 725

570 ml (1 pint) water
1 medium onion
55 g (2 oz) soya mince
140 g (5 oz) tomato purée
1 400 g (14 oz) tin of chopped tomatoes
30 ml (2 tbsp) soy sauce
1.25 – 2.5 ml (1/4 – 1/2 tsp) chilli powder
1 × 450 g (16 oz) tin of red kidney beans
30 ml (2 tbsp) cider vinegar

Measure the water and tip a small amount into a deep saucepan. Place over a high flame and, when simmering, add the finely chopped onion. Sauté the onion for 3 – 5 minutes or until tender.

Add the soya mince and the rest of the water and stir well. Blend in the tomato purée and the chopped tomato. Reduce the heat and add the soy sauce, chilli powder and the beans. Stir well, then cover the pan and leave to simmer for 25 – 30 minutes.

Five minutes before serving, add the vinegar and stir once again. Serve in bowls with a side salad or a slice of Black Bread (page 98).

Shepherdess Pie

SERVES 4 – 6
TOTAL CARBOHYDRATE: 95 g
TOTAL CALORIES: 650

55 g (2 oz) red lentils
55 g (2 oz) soya mince
2.5 ml (¹/2 tsp) freshly ground black pepper
5 ml (1 tsp) mixed sweet dry herbs
710 ml (1¹/4 pints) water
15 ml (1 tbsp) yeast extract
2 medium onions
225 g (¹/2 lb) carrots
225 g (¹/2 lb) Brussels sprouts
225 g (¹/2 lb) potatoes

Wash, rinse and drain the red lentils. In a small bowl, mix the
soya mince, pepper and herbs. Add the drained lentils and stir
the whole together very well. Measure the water and dissolve
the yeast extract in it. Pour this 'gravy' over the lentil and
soya mixture and stir again. Leave to one side.

Peel and slice the onions. Scrub, trim and slice the carrots.
Wash and trim the brussels sprouts then cut each one in half.
Scrub the potatoes and slice them thinly into rounds. (NOTE:
You may find it quicker to slice the vegetables with a food
processor. Keep the potatoes separate from the other vegetables
for the time being).

Mix the vegetables (except the potatoes) in with the lentil
and soya mix. Stir together then tip the mixture into a deep
casserole dish or large baking tin. Arrange the potato slices to
cover the casserole mix.

Cover the dish and bake at 180°C/350°F/Gas Mark 4 for 30
minutes. Remove the cover and bake for a further 10 – 15
minutes. Serve.

Leaf & Lentil Lasagne

SERVES 6 – 8
TOTAL CARBOHYDRATE: 415 g
TOTAL CALORIES: 2280

450 g (1 lb) whole wheat lasagne noodles
225 g ($^1/_2$ lb) fresh spinach
115 g (4 oz) red lentils
2 small onions
1 × 400 g (14 oz) tin of chopped tomatoes
140 g (5 oz) tomato purée
340 ml (12 fl.oz) water
2.5 ml ($^1/_2$ tsp) dried basil
2.5 ml ($^1/_2$ tsp) dried oregano
freshly ground black pepper to taste
1 bunch of fresh parsley
225 g (8 oz) cottage cheese

Bring some water to boil in a deep saucepan and half cook the lasagne noodles in it. Drain and put to one side. Wash, trim and coarsely chop the spinach. Wash and drain the red lentils. Peel and finely chop the onions. Mix the tomatoes, purée and water together in a jug. Add the basil, oregano and black pepper. Wash and finely chop the parsley. Warm the oven to 170°C/325°F/Gas Mark 3.

Arrange two or three lasagne noodles in the bottom of a baking tray. Place a handful of spinach over the noodles. Spoon some of the lentils over the spinach. Place a few slices of onion over the lentils. Sprinkle some chopped parsley over the onions and pour a little of the tomato sauce over the parsley. Spoon a little cottage cheese over the sauce. Repeat the layers two or three times more: noodles, spinach, lentils, onions, parsley, sauce, cheese. Finish with a layer of sauce. Bake for 45 minutes. Serve hot or cold, with salad or steamed vegetables.

Easy Stuffed Peppers

TOTAL CARBOHYDRATE: 55 g
TOTAL CALORIES: 545

30 ml (2 tbsp) yeast extract
285 ml (10 fl.oz) water
2 small onions
55 g (2 oz) soya mince
2.5 ml (¹/2 tsp) freshly ground black pepper
2 medium red peppers
2 medium green peppers
115 g (¹/4 lb) carrots
115 g (¹/4 lb) button mushrooms
25 g (1 oz) fresh parsley
225 g (8 oz) cottage cheese

Dissolve the yeast extract in the water and pour a tiny amount into a frying pan. Peel and finely chop the onions and sauté them in the liquid over a medium flame. Add more liquid, stir in the soya mince and the black pepper. Reduce the heat and cover the pan. Keep over the heat for 5 – 10 minutes, stirring occasionally.

Wash the peppers and slice them in half along their length. Remove the seed cluster and arrange the pepper shells in a baking tray. Scrub, trim and shred the carrots. Clean and quarter the mushrooms. Wash and finely chop the parsley. Stir the carrots, mushrooms and parsley into the soya stuffing. Fill each pepper half with stuffing and top with a spoonful of cottage cheese.

Cover the tray and bake the peppers for 25 minutes at 180°C/350°F/Gas Mark 4. Uncover the tray and bake for a further 5 minutes. Serve immediately with rice or salad – one red, one green half pepper per person.

Stuffed Burgers in Onion Sauce

SERVES 4
TOTAL CARBOHYDRATE: 65 g
TOTAL CALORIES: 545

1 packet of No-Salt VegeBurger dry mix
2.5 ml (1/2 tsp) freshly ground black pepper
25 g (1 oz) tahini
140 ml (5 fl.oz) water
225 g (1/2 lb) button mushrooms
a little whole wheat flour
2 medium onions
3 cloves of garlic (optional)
15 ml (1 tbsp) yeast extract
285 ml (10 fl.oz) water

Blend the VegeBurger mix, black pepper and tahini together in a mixing bowl. Add the water and stir very well. Set to one side for 10 minutes.

Clean and halve the mushrooms. Divide the burger mix into sixteen parts. Roll each part into a ball then place on a floured work surface and roll each ball flat, into a burger. Arrange the sliced mushrooms on to eight of the burgers. Wet the edges of all the burgers and press the eight plain burgers over those covered with mushrooms. Press the edges firmly together and place the stuffed burgers (there should be eight) on a baking tray.

Bake the stuffed burgers at 170°C/325°F/Gas Mark 3 for 15 minutes. Then turn them using a spatula and continue baking for a further 10 minutes. Meanwhile, peel and finely chop the onions and garlic.

Dissolve the yeast extract in the water and pour a little of it into a frying pan. Place over a medium heat and saute the onions and garlic in this liquid. Once they have softened, add the rest of the liquid, cover the pan, reduce the heat and simmer gently for 10 – 15 minutes.

When the burgers are cooked, place them in a warmed serving dish and pour the hot onion sauce over them. Serve with rice, pasta, potatoes or other vegetable dishes.

All-In-One Roast Vegetable Tray

SERVES 4
TOTAL CARBOHYDRATE: 130 g
TOTAL CALORIES: 595

450 g (1 lb) turnips
450 g (1 lb) potatoes
450 g (1 lb) carrots
225 g (1/2 lb) onions
30 ml (2 tbsp) yeast extract
570 ml (1 pint) water
5 ml (1 tsp) dried parsley
2.5 ml (1/2 tsp) dried thyme
2.5 ml (1/2 tsp) dried sage

Scrub, trim and coarsely chop the turnip, potatoes and carrots. Peel and coarsely chop the onions. Arrange these vegetables together in a casserole or baking dish.

Dissolve the yeast extract in the water and stir in the dried herbs. Pour half of this liquid over the vegetables, the other half into a small saucepan. Cover the vegetables and bake at 170°C/325°F/Gas Mark 3 for 40 minutes.

Heat the remaining gravy in the saucepan and pour into a gravy boat for use at the table. Serve the roast vegetables with rice or vegetable cutlet.

Orange & Vegetable Kebabs

SERVES 4

TOTAL CARBOHYDRATE: 25 g

TOTAL CALORIES: 225

2 small onions
1 medium red pepper
1 medium green pepper
115 g (4 oz) button mushrooms
115 g (4 oz) pitted green olives
1 large orange

Peel and quarter the onions. Wash and coarsely chop the peppers. Clean the mushrooms and cut the large ones in half. Drain the olives.

Peel the orange and divide it into segments. Cut each segment in half. Arrange a selection of the vegetables on each of eight skewers (metal or bamboo). Place the kebabs across a baking tray. Grill the kebabs for 2 – 3 minutes, turn or rotate them and grill them for another 2 minutes.

Serve immediately – two kebabs per person –with rice or salad and a sauce of your choice. (Rich Tomato Sauce: page 85; Peanut Sauce: page 91; Fennel Sauce: page 91.)

Cooking Brown Rice

450 g (1 lb) of raw brown rice makes approximately 6 cupsful of cooked rice (the rice trebles in bulk). This is usually enough to serve 4 – 6 people when a sauce or savoury accompanies the rice.

This amount of rice has a total Carbohydrate value of 350 g and a total Calorie value of 1620.

Measure the rice into a mixing bowl and cover with cold water. Now wash the rice by swirling your hand through it and exerting a scrubbing motion. Drain the water and repeat this process three times until the water is fairly clear. Drain the rice and tip into an iron pot.

When cooking rice, the ratio of water to rice is generally 2/1.

Cover the clean rice in the pan with twice its volume in water. Cover the pan and place over a high flame. Bring the water to the boil, then reduce the flame as much as possible and leave to simmer for approximately 50 minutes or until the water is completely absorbed. Keep the pan covered while it cooks, only lifting the lid at the end of the cooking time to check that the rice is finished.

Don't stir the rice at this point, or it may become gummy. If it is still too firm at the end of 50 minutes, boil the kettle and add a little boiling water to the rice. Cover again and cook for another 10 minutes.

Brown rice takes longer to cook than white rice because it is a whole grain. However, it is more nutritious than white, refined rice and has ten times the flavour.

Cooking Beans

Most beans double in bulk once they are cooked.

The carbohydrate and calorie values vary greatly between the different beans but, on a rough average:
the Carbohydrate value per 25 g (1 oz) of *dry beans* is 10 – 15 g and the Calorie value per 25 g (1 oz) of *dry beans* is 70 – 90.

Measure the beans into a mixing bowl and pick them over to remove any stones or unwanted pieces of bean.

Cover the beans with cold water and wash them very well by swirling your hand through them and exerting a scrubbing motion. Pour the water away and repeat this process three times, or until the water is clear. Drain the beans.

Cover the beans with water and leave them to soak overnight or all day while you are at work. Soaking the beans helps to prevent the flatulence that some people suffer from eating beans.

Drain the beans and throw the water away. Tip the beans into an iron pot and cover them with water. Bring them to the boil and simmer with the pan partially covered for 1 – 3 hours, depending on the type of bean you are cooking. The beans must remain covered in water and they must cook until they are easily squashed between your tongue and the top of your mouth. If they are undercooked you will get a stomach ache.

Alternatively, some beans may be pressure cooked. Cover the beans with water, cover the cooker and bring up to pressure. Cook at pressure for 20 – 40 minutes, depending on the type of bean you are cooking. (Please refer to the leaflet accompanying your pressure cooker.)

In both methods, adding a strip of Kombu to the water will help to soften the beans.

Red Lentils and Split Peas do not require soaking or pressure cooking. They do require washing. The red lentils are especially quick to cook and are therefore very useful for a quick, nutritious 'complete protein' meal.

Chickpeas: take 30 minutes in the pressure cooker; 3 hours in the pot.
Kidney Beans: take 30 minutes in the pressure cooker; 1^{1}/2 hours in the pot.
Butter Beans: take 30 minutes in the pressure cooker; 1^{1}/2 hours in the pot.
Soy Beans: take 40 minutes in the pressure cooker; at least 3 hours in the pot.
Black-eyed Beans: take 20 minutes in the pressure cooker; 1 hour in the pot.
Lentils & Split Peas: take 20 minutes in the pressure cooker; 1 hour in the pot.

SAUCES, DRESSINGS & SPREADS

Rich Tomato Sauce

MAKES 285 ml (10 fl.oz)
TOTAL CARBOHYDRATE: 35 g
TOTAL CALORIES: 205

140 ml (5 fl.oz) water
140 ml (5 fl.oz) cider vinegar
60 ml (2 fl.oz) soy sauce
4 large prunes
140 g (5 oz) tomato purée
pinch of ground cloves
2.5 ml (1/2 tsp) ground coriander
5 ml (1 tsp) paprika

Mix the water, vinegar and soy sauce together in a jug. Add the prunes to the liquid and leave to one side. Empty the tomato purée into a small saucepan. Add the spices and blend well, then add the liquid with the softened prunes. Stir well.

Simmer the mixture over a low heat for 20 minutes, keeping it covered except for one or two stirs. Then remove from the heat, press the pip out of each prune, remove the pips and leave the fruit in the sauce.

Serve this sauce hot over pasta, rice, nut loaf, vegetables or as the sauce for barbecue or baked beans.

Tahini Dressing

MAKES 285 ml (10 fl.oz)
TOTAL CARBOHYDRATE: 20 g
TOTAL CALORIES: 270

225 g (8 oz) plain yoghurt
30 ml (2 tbsp) tahini
15 ml (1 tbsp) soy sauce
2.5 ml (1/2 tsp) ground coriander

Mix all the ingredients together in a bowl and stir well. Serve chilled.

Mustard Sauce 1

MAKES 285 ml (10 fl.oz)
TOTAL CARBOHYDRATE: 15 g
TOTAL CALORIES: 175

15 ml (1 tbsp) whole wheat flour
10 ml (2 tsp) dry mustard
15 ml (1 tbsp) margarine
140 ml (5 fl.oz) milk
140 ml (5 fl.oz) water
2.5 ml (1/2 tsp) freshly ground black pepper

Mix the flour and dry mustard together in a cup.

Melt the margarine in a small saucepan then sprinkle the flour mixture into the pan and stir well to form a thick paste, or roux.

Keep the roux over the heat and gradually add the milk and water, stirring all the while. Add water if a more liquid consistency is needed.

Add the pepper and stir continuously to form a smooth, thick sauce. Serve immediately.

Mustard Sauce 2

MAKES 110 ml (4 fl.oz)
TOTAL CARBOHYDRATE: negligible
TOTAL CALORIES: 145

3 cloves of garlic
30 ml (1 fl.oz) oil
90 ml (3 fl.oz) cider vinegar
10 ml (2 tsp) wet mustard
2.5 ml (1/2 tsp) dried mint

Chop or crush the garlic into a jam jar. Add the other ingredients, cover the jar, and shake very well. Serve over a salad or simple steamed vegetables.

Yoghurt Sauce 1

MAKES 285 ml (10 fl.oz)
TOTAL CARBOHYDRATE: 20 g
TOTAL CALORIES: 160

285 g (10 oz) plain yoghurt
30 ml (2 tbsp) chopped chives or 2 spring onions
2.5 ml (1/2 tsp) paprika

Empty the yoghurt into a small bowl. Chop the chives or spring onions and stir into the yoghurt. Next sprinkle the paprika over the yoghurt and stir gently to give a swirled or 'marble' effect. Allow to chill for 10 minutes before serving.

Use as a dip for raw vegetables, a dressing for salads or drop a spoonful on to your favourite soup just before serving.

Yoghurt Sauce 2

MAKES 285 ml (10 fl.oz)
TOTAL CARBOHYDRATE: 20 g
TOTAL CALORIES: 175

285 g (10 oz) plain yoghurt
10 ml (2 tsp) wet mustard
5 ml (1 tsp) dill seed

Stir all the ingredients together in a small bowl. If a thinner sauce is preferred, add 15 ml (1 tbsp) vinegar. Serve chilled over a salad or baked potato.

Mint Vinaigrette

MAKES 90 ml (3 fl.oz)
TOTAL CARBOHYDRATE: 15 g
TOTAL CALORIES: 40

90 ml (3 fl.oz) cider vinegar
5 ml (1 tsp) honey
5 ml (1 tsp) dried mint
2.5 ml (1/2 tsp.) freshly ground black pepper.

Mix all the ingredients together in a jar and shake well. Pour over a salad or simple steamed vegetables.

Simple Yoghurt Dip

MAKES 140 ml (5 fl.oz)
TOTAL CARBOHYDRATE: 15 g
TOTAL CALORIES: 100

140 g (5 oz) plain yoghurt
1 – 2.5 ml (1/4 – 1/2 tsp) paprika
5 ml (1 tsp) tomato purée

Mix all the ingredients together in a small bowl and whisk well. Serve as a dip for raw vegetables, as a dressing for salads or float a spoonful in a bowl of your favourite soup.

Simple Lemon Dressing

MAKES 90 ml (3 fl.oz)
TOTAL CARBOHYDRATE: negligible
TOTAL CALORIES: 30

juice of 2 lemons
2.5 ml (1/2 tsp) freshly ground black pepper
15 ml (1 tbsp) chopped fresh parsley

Squeeze the lemon juice into a jug and add the ground pepper. Wash and finely chop the fresh parsley and stir into the lemon juice. Leave to stand in the jug for 10 – 15 minutes, then pour over individual portions of salad.

Very Own Catsup

MAKES 250 ml (8 fl.oz)
TOTAL CARBOHYDRATE: 15 g
TOTAL CALORIES: 110

140 g (5 oz) tomato purée
30 ml (2 tbsp) soy sauce
60 ml (4 tbsp) vinegar
2 cloves of garlic (optional)
a pinch of chilli powder

Mix all the ingredients together in a bowl. If using garlic, crush it rather than chop it. Stir well and allow to stand for 30 – 60 minutes before serving.

Banana & Mustard Chutney

MAKES 90 ml (3 fl.oz)
TOTAL CARBOHYDRATE: 25 g
TOTAL CALORIES: 110

2 very ripe bananas
30 ml (2 tbsp) sharp wet mustard

Mash the bananas in a small bowl. Stir in the mustard to an even consistency. Serve with rice dishes, steamed vegetables, baked potatoes, or just about anything!

Hot Peanut Sauce

SERVES 4 – 6
TOTAL CARBOHYDRATE: 10 g
TOTAL CALORIES: 180

1 clove of garlic
15 ml (1 tbsp) unsalted crunchy peanut butter
15 ml (1 tbsp) soy sauce
juice of 1 lemon
140 ml (5 fl.oz) water

Peel and finely chop the garlic into a small saucepan. Add the peanut butter and place over a medium flame, stirring often. When the garlic begins to soften, add the soy sauce. Stir well then add the lemon juice. Again, stir well and gradually add the water. Reduce the heat and keep covered for 5 – 10 minutes.

Serve with any rice or vegetable dish, or vegetable or nut loaf.

Fennel Sauce

SERVES 6 – 8
TOTAL CARBOHYDRATE: 15 g
TOTAL CALORIES: 60

1 large sweet fennel
1 green eating apple
juice of 1 lemon
2.5 ml (1/2 tsp) ground coriander

Wash and trim the fennel and cut into small chunks. Place in a food processor. Quarter and core the apple and place in the food processor. Add the lemon juice and the coriander to the processor and purée all the ingredients together to a fine consistency.

Serve chilled with raw vegetables, in soups or as a dressing to a salad.

Fruit Chutney

SERVES 4 – 6
TOTAL CARBOHYDRATE: 75 g
TOTAL CALORIES: 315

115 g (4 oz) raisins or sultanas
60 ml (2 fl.oz) water
15 ml (1 tbsp) grated fresh ginger
1 very ripe banana
juice of 1 lemon
30 – 60 ml (2 – 4 tbsp) chopped fresh coriander

Rinse and pick over the raisins then place them in a small saucepan with the water. Bring to a boil and simmer, covered, for 5 minutes. Grate the ginger and mash it with the banana in a small bowl. Add to the ingredients in the pan, stir well and cover again.

Squeeze the lemon and stir the chopped coriander into it. Add these to the ingredients in the pan also. Stir well and cook a further 5 minutes over a very low heat. Serve immediately or allow to cool and then chill the chutney for later use.

Poppy Seed Sauce

MAKES 570 ml (1 pint)
TOTAL CARBOHYDRATE: 25 g
TOTAL CALORIES: 255

15 ml (1 tbsp) margarine
15 ml (1 tbsp) poppy seed
15 ml (1 tbsp) whole wheat flour
5 ml (1 tsp) ground coriander
285 ml (10 fl.oz) milk
285 ml (10 fl.oz) water

Melt the margarine in a small saucepan over a low heat. Add the poppy seed and sauté for 2 – 3 minutes, stirring constantly. Mix the flour and coriander together then sprinkle them over the margarine to make a smooth paste, or roux.

Put the milk and water together in a jug and gradually add the liquid to the roux, stirring constantly to maintain a smooth consistency. Add more water if a more liquid sauce is desired.

Serve immediately over green vegetables, baked potatoes, or pasta.

Mushroom Pâté

SERVES 4 – 6
TOTAL CARBOHYDRATE: 115 g
TOTAL CALORIES: 590

450 g (1 pound) button mushrooms
225 g (8 oz) cooked brown rice
55 g (2 oz) fresh breadcrumbs
juice of 1 lemon
2.5 ml (¹/2 tsp) freshly ground black pepper

Clean the mushrooms and place them in a food processor with the rice, breadcrumbs, lemon juice and pepper. Purée to an even consistency, adding a little water if necessary.

Spoon into a serving dish, press the pâté down firmly and chill before serving.

Easy Lentil Pâté

SERVES 6 – 8
TOTAL CARBOHYDRATE: 185 g
TOTAL CALORIES: 1000

225 g (8 oz) dried red lentils
570 ml (1 pint) water
pinch of salt
50 g (2 oz) porridge oats
50 g (2 oz) rice flakes
5 ml (1 tsp) ground black pepper or paprika
2.5 ml (¹/2 tsp) ground ginger

Wash lentils and drain. Add the clean water and salt and bring to a soft boil. Cover and simmer for 30 minutes, stirring often. Add oats, rice flakes, pepper and ginger and simmer for another 5 – 10 minutes.

Remove from the heat and spoon into a serving dish. Allow the pâté to cool, then chill or serve immediately.

Red Bean Paste

SERVES 4
TOTAL CARBOHYDRATE: 75 g
TOTAL CALORIES: 340

115 g (4 oz) dried kidney or pinto beans
2 small onions
2.5 ml (1/2 tsp) chilli powder
15 ml (1 tbsp) soy sauce
30 ml (2 tbsp) cider vinegar
300 – 400 ml (10 – 14 fl.oz) water

Wash, soak, rinse and pressure cook the beans. Chop the onions and sauté with the chilli powder in the soy sauce and vinegar.

Add the cooked beans and mash them slightly as you gradually add the water. Aim for a thick paste. If you prefer a smoother texture, run the paste through a hand mouli or food processor. Serve hot or allow to cool and chill in its serving dish.

Mung Bean Dip

SERVES 2 – 4
TOTAL CARBOHYDRATE: 30 g
TOTAL CALORIES: 230

225 g (8 oz) cooked mung beans
140 g (5 oz) plain yoghurt
2.5 ml (1/2 tsp) dried mint
salt to taste

Measure all the ingredients into a bowl and mash them together with a fork. For a smoother texture, use a blender. Serve in sandwiches, on crackers, for stuffing vegetables or as a dip for raw celery and carrots.

BREADS & BREAKFASTS

Sourdough Bread

MAKES 2 LOAVES
TOTAL CARBOHYDRATE: 615 g
TOTAL CALORIES: 2955

The Starter:
45 ml (3 tbsp) plain flour
75 ml (5 tbsp) water

Stir the flour and water into a paste. Cover the bowl first with
a paper towel and then a small plate and leave for 2 – 3 days.
It will become more liquid and bubbly.

The Bread:
1 kg (2 lb) whole wheat flour
the sourdough starter
710 – 850 ml (1^1/4 – 1^1/2 pints) water

Stir all the ingredients together, knead the dough and then shape
it into loaf tins or rounds on a baking tray.

Allow to rise, covered, for 12 hours or overnight. Uncover
and bake at 160°C/200°F/ Gas Mark 3 for 40 minutes. Allow
to cool on a rack.

Black Bread

MAKES 2 LOAVES
TOTAL CARBOHYDRATE: 650 g
TOTAL CALORIES: 3060

850 ml (1¹/2 pints) tepid water
30 ml (2 tbsp) molasses
15 ml (1 tbsp) dried yeast
450 g (1 lb) rye flour
450 g (1 lb) whole wheat flour

Measure half the water into a jug and dissolve the molasses in it. Then add the dried yeast to the liquid, stir well and leave to work for 5 – 10 minutes.

Mix the rye and wheat flours together in a large bowl.

When the yeast has worked, stir it into the flour mixture with a large wooden spoon. Gradually add more of the water, stirring constantly.

When the dough is too thick to stir, use your hands and knead it to a firm consistency. The amount of water needed will vary – add more than the stated amount if the dough is too dry, and be prepared to add more flour if the dough becomes sticky and unmanageable.

When you have kneaded the dough for about 5 minutes, form it into a ball in the bowl, cover the bowl and leave in a warm place to rise for 45 minutes.

Knead the dough again and shape into loaves. Place them in an oiled bread tin and, again, leave to rise in a warm place for 30 minutes.

Bake at 170°C/325°F/Gas Mark 3 for 35 minutes.

Healthy Pumpkin Bread

MAKES 1 LARGE LOAF
TOTAL CARBOHYDRATE: 315 g
TOTAL CALORIES: 1570

340 g (12 (oz) whole wheat flour
10 ml (2 tsp) baking powder
2.5 ml (¹/2 tsp) ground cinnamon
2.5 ml (¹/2 tsp) ground nutmeg or allspice
115 g (4 oz) raisins or sultanas
285 g (10 oz) tinned, prepared pumpkin
2 medium eggs
140 ml (5 fl.oz) water

Warm the oven to 170°C/325°F/Gas Mark 3. Lightly oil a loaf tin. Measure the flour, baking powder and spices into a mixing bowl and blend together. Add the raisins and stir well.

In a separate bowl, mix the pumpkin, eggs and water and whisk briskly to a light, airy consistency. Add this to the dry mixture and stir well for 2 –3 minutes.

Spoon the mixture into the loaf tin and bake for 45 minutes. Cool on a wire rack and serve the same day with margarine or sugarless jam.

Raisin Bread Roll

SERVES 4 – 6
TOTAL CARBOHYDRATE: 245 g
TOTAL CALORIES: 1190

225 g (8 oz) whole wheat flour
10 ml (2 tsp) baking powder
50 g (2 oz) margarine
140 ml (5 fl.oz) water
115 g (4 oz) raisins
pinch of cinnamon
pinch of ground cloves
15 ml (1 tbsp) honey

Mix flour and baking powder together in a bowl and cut in the margarine. Add the water and stir well. Roll the dough into a rectangle on a lightly floured board to approximately 1/2" thickness.

Sprinkle the raisins and spices over the dough and trickle the honey over the raisins. Roll the rectangle, seal the edges and bake at 170°C/325°F/Gas Mark 3 for 30 – 40 minutes. Cool, slice and serve.

Breakfast Fruit Bowl

SERVES 2
TOTAL CARBOHYDRATE: 195 g
TOTAL CALORIES: 810

50 g (2 oz) dried dates
50 g (2 oz) dried figs
1 eating apple
1 orange
50 g (2 oz) raisins
285 ml (10 fl.oz) orange juice
50 g (2 oz) rolled oats
2.5 ml (1/2 tsp) cinnamon

Wash and chop the dates, figs, and apple. Peel and slice the orange and mix all the fruit with the raisins and orange juice in a large bowl.

Add the oats and cinnamon and stir well. Allow to sit for 10 minutes then serve in small bowls —with a dollop of yoghurt if desired.

Quick Porridge Royale

SERVES 2
TOTAL CARBOHYDRATE: 145 g
TOTAL CALORIES: 640

115 g (4 oz) porridge oats
50g (2 oz) raisins [32 g CHO/120 cal]
570 ml (1 pint) water
4 small pitted dates [20 g CHO/80 cal]
1 eating apple

Measure the oats into a saucepan with the raisins. Pour the water over, stir and place over a low flame. Stir frequently. Wash and finely chop the dates and the apple.

When the porridge is quite thick, add the fruit and stir well. Serve hot. To reduce either the calorie or carbohydrate count, use *either* the raisins *or* the dates, but not both.

Apple Dilly

SERVES 4
TOTAL CARBOHYDRATE: 80 g
TOTAL CALORIES: 370

900 g (2 lb) cooking apples
juice of 1 lemon
2.5 ml (1/2 tsp) ground cinnamon
140 g (5 oz) plain yoghurt

Wash, quarter and core the apples.

Chop them quite finely into an enamel saucepan with the lemon juice. Place the pan over a medium flame and stir the softening apples often.

Add the cinnamon and stir frequently.

When the apple has cooked to a soft, mushy texture remove the pan from the heat and ladle the hot dilly into bowls.

Top each serving with a little yoghurt and serve immediately.

Easy Fruit Pudding

SERVES 2 – 4
TOTAL CARBOHYDRATE: 95 g
TOTAL CALORIES: 435

225 (8 oz) cooked brown rice
140 ml (5 fl.oz) milk
450 g (1 lb) fresh blackberries

Measure the rice and milk into a saucepan and stir well.

Place over a medium heat and, stirring often, bring the pudding to a simmer. Allow the rice to soften and thicken, then add the berries. Stir well and serve.

Gourmet Melon

SERVES 2
TOTAL CARBOHYDRATE: 70 g
TOTAL CALORIES: 425

1 *whole honeydew melon*
2 *satsumas* or *mandarins*
55 g (2 oz) *raisins* or *sultanas*
140 ml (5 fl.oz) *orange juice*
25 g (1 oz) *dessicated coconut*

Cut the melon in half and scoop out the seeds. Peel the satsumas and divide them into segments. Measure the raisins into a bowl and add the satsumas to them.

Pour the orange juice into the bowl and stir well. Leave to soak for 5 – 10 minutes, then add the coconut. Stir again and spoon the mixture into the melon halves. Serve immediately with ground nutmeg or cinnamon at hand, or chill and serve.

Baked Omelette

SERVES 2 – 4
TOTAL CARBOHYDRATE: average 100 g
TOTAL CALORIES: average 650

3 (size 3) free range eggs
285 ml (10 fl.oz) milk
2.5 ml (¹/2 tsp) mixed sweet dry herbs
freshly ground black pepper to taste
450 g (1 lb) pre-cooked, tinned or frozen vegetables i.e. peas, carrots,
sweet corn, cooked potatoes, broccoli

Whisk the eggs and milk together in a mixing bowl. Add the
dry herbs and pepper and whisk again to a light frothiness. Use
a fork to stir in your blend of vegetables so that they are all
coated in the egg mixture.

Warm the oven to 170°C/325°F/Gas Mark 3 and lightly oil
a flan dish. Pour the omelette mixture into the flan dish and
cover with foil. Bake for 25 minutes then remove the foil and
bake for a further 5 – 10 minutes. Slice into halves or quarters
and serve hot.

DRINKS & DESSERTS

Lemonade With Orange Cubes

SERVES 4
TOTAL CARBOHYDRATE: 35 g
TOTAL CALORIES: 220

270 ml (¹/2 pint) orange juice
6 lemons
1 litre (2 pints) water
2 sprigs of mint

Pour orange juice into an ice cube tray and freeze. Wash and slice the lemons into a deep bowl. Boil the water and pour over the lemons. Allow to cool. When tepid, add the clean mint. Stir well, allow to cool further and add the frozen orange cubes just before serving.

Citrus Tea

SERVES 2
TOTAL CARBOHYDRATE: negligible
TOTAL CALORIES: 10

570 ml (1 pint) boiling water
2 slices of lemon
2 slices of orange
1 sprig of fresh mint

Boil the water and use a little to warm a tea pot that has not
been used for normal tea. Add the citrus slices and clean mint
to the pot. Pour the boiling water over, stir, cover and allow
to 'brew' for 5 minutes. This is a very refreshing drink which
also stimulates your digestion.

Thick Pumpkin Milkshake

SERVES 2
TOTAL CARBOHYDRATE: 60 g
TOTAL CALORIES: 370

225 g (8 oz) tinned pumpkin
570 ml (1 pint) milk
2.5 ml (1/2 tsp) ground allspice
140 g (5 oz) plain yoghurt

Measure the pumpkin into a saucepan and add the milk to it.
Stir well and place over a low flame. Simmer very gently for 5
minutes, stirring constantly. Add the allspice to the mixture,
stir well and allow to cool.

When cool, stir in the yoghurt. Pour into large tumblers and
chill for 30 – 60 minutes. Serve very cold.

Almond Milk

SERVES 2 – 4
TOTAL CARBOHYDRATE: 25 g
TOTAL CALORIES: 560

115 g (4 oz) whole shelled almonds
850 ml (1.5 pints) very cold water

Measure the almonds into a mixing bowl and cover them with tepid water. Leave them to soak overnight, or for 8 – 12 hours. Drain and rinse the soaked almonds and remove their skins.

Put the peeled almonds in a food processor with the 850 ml of water. Purée to a very fine, very smooth consistency.

Strain the milk through cheesecloth or a paper coffee filter into a jug. Allow 10 – 15 minutes for the milk to finish filtering. Serve this pure white milk immediately. Use the almond pulp in baking if you wish.

Nutmeg & Watercress Tea

SERVES 2
TOTAL CARBOHYDRATE: negligible
TOTAL CALORIES: 25

1 bunch of watercress
half of a whole nutmeg or 2.5 ml (1/2 tsp) ground nutmeg
850 ml (1.5 pints) water

Wash, trim and chop the watercress and place in an enamel saucepan with the nutmeg and water. Bring to the boil, then reduce the heat, cover the pan and simmer for 10 minutes. Strain the 'tea' into cups and serve.

Baked Citrus Compote

SERVES 4
TOTAL CARBOHYDRATE: 75 g
TOTAL CALORIES: 410

2 grapefruit
2 oranges
1 lemon
50 g (2 oz) raisins
For the Sauce:
140 ml (5 fl.oz) red wine
6 whole cloves
a piece of cinnamon stick

Carefully peel and section the fruits and place in a shallow casserole dish. Add the raisins and stir the fruits together. Prepare the sauce by simply mixing the wine and spices together in a jug. Pour over the fruit and allow it to soak for 10 minutes. Stir again.

Warm the oven to 170°C/325°F/Gas Mark 3. Cover the compote and bake for 20 minutes. Serve immediately, pouring a little of the sauce over each serving.

Banana Splitz

SERVES 4
TOTAL CARBOHYDRATE: 65 g
TOTAL CALORIES: 430

4 large bananas
115 g (4 oz) gooseberries or *loganberries* or *redcurrants* or *a mixture*
225 g (8 oz) plain yoghurt
28 g (1 oz) chopped nuts

Peel the bananas and slice them in half along their length. Place each split banana on its individual serving dish. Fill each split banana with one-quarter of the fruit you have chosen. For each serving, spoon one-quarter of the yoghurt over the fruit. Sprinkle a tiny amount of chopped nuts over the yoghurt.

Chill the 'splitz' until you are ready to serve them. Garnish with a paper umbrella!

Nutty Yoghurt Dessert

SERVES 2
TOTAL CARBOHYDRATE: 40 g
TOTAL CALORIES: 370

200 g (7 oz) plain yoghurt
2.5 ml (1/2 tsp) ground coriander
50 g (2 oz) chestnut purée
28 g (1 oz) chopped nuts

Measure the yoghurt into a small bowl and stir in the ground coriander.

Add the chestnut purée to the yoghurt and use a fork, then a spoon, to work the whole to an even consistency.

Spoon the mixture into two serving dishes and chill until you are ready to serve them. Sprinkle half of the chopped nuts over each serving.

Spicy Oat Cake

SERVES 4 – 6
TOTAL CARBOHYDRATE: 150 g
TOTAL CALORIES: 835

55 g (2 oz) raisins or sultanas
285 ml (10 fl.oz) water
15 ml (1 tbsp) oil
55 g (2 oz) whole wheat flour
115 g (4 oz) rolled oats
2.5 ml ($^{1}/_{2}$ tsp) ground cinnamon
1.25 ml ($^{1}/_{4}$ tsp) ground cloves
7.5 ml ($1^{1}/_{2}$ tsp) baking powder

Measure the raisins into a small bowl and pour the water and oil over them. Stir once, then leave them to soak. Mix the remaining, dry ingredients together in a mixing bowl. Stir well and set aside.

Warm the oven to 170°C/325°F/Gas Mark 3 and lightly oil a 20 cm (8 inch) cake tin. Stir the soaked raisins and the liquid into the dry mix. Stir very well, adding a little more water if necessary to give a smooth, moist batter. Spoon the batter into the cake tin, spread evenly to the corners and bake for 25 –30 minutes. Cool for 15 minutes, then remove from the tin and cool on a rack.

Banana & Yoghurt Mousse

SERVES 4
TOTAL CARBOHYDRATE: 70 g
TOTAL CALORIES: 420

2 ripe bananas
450 g (1 lb) plain yoghurt
40 g (1.5 oz) Allbran cereal

Peel bananas and purée them with the yoghurt. Stir the Allbran into the purée and spoon into four dessert dishes.

Place the servings in the freezer until they are nearly firm —you should be able to push a spoon into them with little effort. Serve immediately.

Cinnamon Orange Rice Pudding

SERVES 4
TOTAL CARBOHYDRATE: 225 g
TOTAL CALORIES: 990

140 ml (5 fl.oz) fresh orange juice
55 g (2 oz) raisins
225 g (8 oz) short-grained brown rice
425 ml (15 fl.oz) water
2.5 ml (1/2 tsp) ground cinnamon

Measure the orange juice into a small bowl and soak the raisins in it. Wash and drain the rice. Add to the water in a saucepan and bring to the boil. Reduce the heat, cover the pan and simmer the rice for 30 – 40 minutes. It should become very soft and sticky.

When most of the water is absorbed, add the orange juice and raisins and stir well. Cover the pan and simmer a further 5 minutes. Stir in the cinnamon, spoon the pudding into its serving dish(es) and serve immediately or cover, allow to cool then chill before serving.

Almond Sandies

MAKES 24 BISCUITS
TOTAL CARBOHYDRATE: 150 g
TOTAL CALORIES: 1050

225 g (8 oz) whole wheat flour
25 g (1 oz) ground almonds
7.5 ml (1.5 tsp) baking powder
55 g (2 oz) margarine
5 ml (1 tsp) natural almond essence
140 ml (5 fl.oz) water

Measure the flour, ground almonds and baking powder into a mixing bowl and stir well. Measure the margarine and cut into the dry mixture until an even consistency is reached. Add the almond essence and the water and work the dough to an evenly moist paste. Use a fork first; then a spoon or your hands. Warm the oven to 180°C/350°F/Gas Mark 4.

Roll the dough into approximately 24 walnut-sized balls and arrange these on a baking tray. Then press the balls of dough flat using the bottom of a glass tumbler. Dip the glass in water to prevent the dough sticking. Bake for 12 – 15 minutes. Cool on wire racks.

Bake 'n Take Bars

MAKES 1 DOZEN
TOTAL CARBOHYDRATE: 220 g
TOTAL CALORIES: 1455

225 g (8 oz) whole wheat flour
55 g (2 oz) rolled oats
55 g (2 oz) shredded coconut
25 g (1 oz) fructose (optional)
5 ml (1 tsp) baking powder
2.5 ml (1/2 tsp) ground cinnamon or allspice
15 ml (1 tbsp) oil
5 ml (1 tsp) natural vanilla essence
140 ml (5 fl.oz) water

Warm the oven to 160°C/300F/Gas Mark 3 and lightly oil a 20 cm (8 inch) cake tin. Mix the first six ingredients together in a mixing bowl. Add the oil, essence and water to the dry mix and stir very well. Spoon the batter evenly into the cake tin and bake for 25 minutes. Allow to cool, then slice and serve.

Marbled Cherry & Carob Cake

SERVES 6 – 8
TOTAL CARBOHYDRATE: 210 g
TOTAL CALORIES: 1180

115 g (4 oz) frozen or *unsweetened tinned cherries*
285 ml (10 fl.oz) water
225 g (8 oz) whole wheat flour
7.5 ml (1.5 tsp) baking powder
55 g (2 oz) carob powder
85 g (3 oz) margarine

Put the cherries in a bowl and measure the water into a jug. Pour 100 ml (3.5 fl.oz) of the water over the cherries and set both to one side.

Measure the flour and divide it evenly between two small mixing bowls (115 g/4 oz in each). Sprinkle half of the baking powder into each bowl.

Add all the carob powder to one bowl. Stir both mixtures separately. Divide the margarine evenly between the two bowls and cut it into the dry mixes using a fork or knife. Work it to an even consistency. Now tip the water in the jug into the bowl which contains the carob mixture. Tip the cherries and their liquid into the other bowl. Stir both mixtures very well.

Warm the oven to 170°C/325°F/Gas Mark 3. Lightly oil a deep cake tin. Scrape the carob batter into the cherry batter and **very gently** fold the two batters together. Spoon the batter into the cake tin and bake for 25 – 30 minutes. Cool for 10 minutes in the tin, then remove and cool on a wire rack.

PART THREE

EATING FOR A GOOD LIFE

NOT JUST FOR DIABETICS!

In the first section of this book, I mentioned the dietary recommendations being made to the whole population. Among these are the low fat, high fibre guidelines recommended for diabetics. There are many reasons for these recommendations being extended to the general population.

The fairly simple expedient of reducing fat intake (especially saturated, animal fat) and of increasing fibre intake can significantly reduce the incidence of obesity, coronary heart disease, hypertension, certain cancers, and diabetes. So while you may be too late to prevent diabetes in yourself or someone close to you, you may minimize the complications of diabetes which can shorten life.

If you have children you can greatly reduce their risk of succumbing to one or more of these life-threatening disorders by improving their diet – now. That makes sense, doesn't it? A sort of edible life insurance policy.

So your special diabetic needs aren't so special after all –they will benefit everyone in your family. There is no need to prepare two separate meals: one traditional, one diabetic. You'll be doing yourself and everyone in your family a very long term, health-giving favour if you help them adhere to a high fibre, low fat diet from now on.

Most of the recipes in this collection are enough for 4 people. You can combine one or two dishes in a meal, make one to go alongside your own creation, or even use an old recipe –but substituting the high fat, low fibre ingredients with healthier products. For instance, *Shepherdess Pie* on page 76 takes an old idea and adds a soya mince substitute; *Leaf & Lentil*

Lasagne and *Stuffed Burgers in Onion Sauce* make similar changes.

There is a great opportunity here for you to throw out dull habits, old routines and be creative and have fun instead. Here are some suggestions for dishes that go well together:

SUNDAY LUNCH MENU

Orange & Asparagus Salad
Yoghurt Sauce 2
Nutless Hot 'N Cold Loaf
All in One Roast Vegetable Tray
Leek & Brussels Sprouts Stir-Fry
Banana Splitz
Citrus 'Tea'

PICNIC OR BARBECUE MENU

Radish & Butter Bean Salad
Potato Salad
Rustic Baked Beans
Mexican Tostadas
Orange & Vegetable Kebabs
Very Own Catsup
Mustard Sauce 2
Lemonade with Orange Cubes

ORIENTAL FLAVOUR MENU

Pea & Coriander Soup
Scented Rice
Aduki Beans & Bamboo Shoots Savoury
Hot Arame & Broccoli Salad
Carrot & Spring Onion Sauté
Banana & Mustard Chutney
Hot Peanut Sauce
Nutmeg & Watercress 'Tea'

Cold Orange & Chestnut Soup
Easy Stuffed Peppers
Sweet Potato Bake
Ladies' Fingers Savoury
Easy Lentil Pâté
Almond Milk
Gourmet Melon

WORDS ON INGREDIENTS

Some of the ingredients listed in the recipes may be new to you. However, all of them are readily available either in supermarkets or in the increasingly common whole food shops. Here are just a few explained:

Arame – is a seaweed with a very curly, lacey texture. It is delicious and not at all fishy!

Branded Diabetic Products – I don't use them. They are expensive and not always better for you. Do it yourself is much more fun.

Kombu – is another seaweed. This one isn't actually eaten, but is used to thicken soups and stews, soften beans while cooking, and to add a very subtle buttery flavour to broths and sauces. It is always optional.

Margarine – I always use a low fat, non-dairy margarine.

Miso – made from the soy bean. This is a fermented paste which may be used instead of yeast extract. Try a spoonful on toast.

Oil – nothing unusual about this, but do avoid buying oil which just says 'vegetable oil' and purchase a named oil instead. They are no more expensive and better for you. For instance, safflower oil, corn oil, sunflower oil or soybean oil.

Soya Milk – is made from the soy bean. It is easy to find and a really tasty alternative to cow's milk. Use it in the same way and pass the word to people with eczema – they might be allergic to cow's milk.

Soya Mince – this is yet another soy bean product made to resemble the look and texture of mince beef.

Soy Sauce – if you are in a whole food shop, Tamari and Shoyu are natural forms of soy sauce.

Tempeh – also a soy bean product (what a wonderful plant!).

This is a block of fermented beans which you will buy frozen from a whole food shop. Don't pull a face at the look of it until you've tried the recipe. Delicious!

Tofu – this is a cheese made from soya milk. It comes either soft or firm and is usually packed in water (some varieties are dried). I use the soft variety instead of yoghurt, the firm variety instead of cheese. Many supermarkets and all whole food shops have this on their shelves now.

Tortillas – these are round, flat cornmeal crispbreads available in many supermarkets.

VegeBurger Mix – this is a meat-free burger mix sold in a foil packet by the Realeat Company. It is an excellent, all natural basis for many traditional dishes, as well as some that you haven't thought of yet. Available in supermarkets.

Yeast Extract – there are so many varieties on the market now, read the labels and pick one that is low in salt.

ANOTHER WORD . . . ON EQUIPMENT

Most of the recipes in this collection are fairly quick to prepare. But some of the labour-saving equipment on the market really does put an end to the 'slave' part of leaning over the kitchen stove. Other equipment is better for being very traditional. Here is a list of my preferences.

Iron pots – if you keep these well oiled to prevent rust, they will add to the iron in your diet every time you cook with them. Aluminium is out because you actually get some of that in your cooking as well - but this time it's *not* good for you. Enamel pots are very good too, though no added iron.

Pressure Cooker – a real time saver when you cook beans. Buy one that is stainless steel. (See page 82 for instructions on cooking beans.)

Food Processor – apart from the noise, these things are as good as having your own kitchen maid. They make *very* short work of shredding, slicing, grating and, of course, puréeing. If I really can't face the noise, or if I'm not in a hurry, then I chop and slice in the normal way, with pleasure.

Mouli – one of those hand-turned sieves that rests on a bowl or pan and pushes soups and jams and sauces through a sloping, perforated blade. You probably know what I mean -it is difficult to describe!

Universal Steamer – this is a perforated metal basket that adjusts to fit into almost any size pan. Place your vegetables in the basket, a bit of water under the basket, cover the pan and steam away.

AND A FINAL WORD ON FURTHER READING & ORGANIZATIONS TO CONTACT

The Diabetes Handbook: Insulin Dependent Diabetes by Dr. John L. Day; Thorsons Publishing Group in collaboration with The British Diabetic Association, 1986.

The Diabetes Handbook: Non-Insulin Dependent Diabetes by Dr. John L.Day; Thorsons Publishing Group in collaboration with The British Diabetic Association, 1986.

Countdown a publication from The British Diabetic Association to guide consumers regarding the calorie and carbohydrate content of manufactured foods.

Why You Don't Need Meat by Peter Cox; Thorsons Publishing Group, 1986

Vegan Nutrition – by Gill Langley; The Vegan Society, 1988, 33–35 George Street, Oxford OX1 2AX, telephone: 0865-722166.

Laurel's Kitchen: A Handbook for Vegetarian Cookery and Nutrition by Laurel Robertson, Carol Flinders and Bronwen Godfrey, Routledge and Kegan Paul, London 1979.

The British Diabetic Association, 10 Queen Anne Street, London W1M OBD, telephone 01-323-1531.

Index